HOME CARE AIDE INSERVICE TRAINING MODULE: SAFETY

For all their patience, understanding, and support,
we dedicate this book to our families.

I will always be grateful to my mother and sisters for their neverending love.
In loving memory of my father who taught me that I could achieve anything
with dedication and hard work. Especially to Phil, thank you for
being my strength and my love.

Jackie Nasso

To my mother, my best friend, for all her unconditional love and support.
To my father, for his wisdom, love, and guidance. To my wonderful husband,
who has helped me grow and become the person I am today.

Lisa Celia

For every page of this book, we thank everyone who could not be mentioned.

HOME CARE AIDE INSERVICE TRAINING MODULE: SAFETY

Jackie Nasso, MPA, BSN, RN
Lisa Celia, BSN, RN

THOMSON
DELMAR LEARNING

Australia   Canada   Mexico   Singapore   Spain   United Kingdom   United States

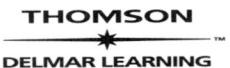

Home Care Aide Inservice Training Module: Safety
by Jackie Nasso and Lisa Celia

Vice President, Health Care Business Unit:
William Brottmiller

Editorial Director:
Cathy L. Esperti

Acquisitions Editor:
Marah Bellegarde

Editorial Assistant:
Jadin Babin-Kavanaugh

Marketing Director:
Jennifer McAvey

Marketing Coordinator:
Kimberly Duffy

Production Editor:
Anne Sherman

COPYRIGHT © 2005 by Thomson Delmar Learning. Thomson and Delmar Learning are trademarks used herein under license.

Printed in Canada
1 2 3 4 5 6 XXX 09 08 07 06 05

For more information, contact Thomson Delmar Learning, 5 Maxwell Drive, Clifton Park, NY 12065
Or find us on the World Wide Web at
http://www.delmarlearning.com

ALL RIGHTS RESERVED. No part of this work covered by the copyright hereon may be reproduced or used in any form or by any means—graphic, electronic, or mechanical, including photocopying, recording, taping, Web distribution or information storage and retrieval systems—without the written permission of the publisher.

For permission to use material from this text or product, contact us by
Tel (800) 730-2214
Fax (800) 730-2215
www.thomsonrights.com

Library of Congress Cataloging-in-Publication Data
Nasso, Jackie.
  Home care aide inservice training module. Safety / Jackie Nasso, Lisa Celia.
    p. cm.
  Also issued as part of a binder entitled: Home care aide : inservice training modules.
  Includes bibliographical references.
  ISBN 1-4018-9757-6 (alk. paper)
  1. Home health aides--Training of. 2. Home health aides--Study and teaching. 3. Home care services. I. Title: Safety. II. Nasso, Jackie. Home care aide. III. Celia. Lisa. IV. Title.
RA645.3.N374 2005
362.14--dc22   2005041857

Notice to the Reader

Publisher does not warrant or guarantee any of the products described herein or perform any independent analysis in connection with any of the product information contained herein. Publisher does not assume, and expressly disclaims, any obligation to obtain and include information other than that provided to it by the manufacturer.

The reader is expressly warned to consider and adopt all safety precautions that might be indicated by the activities described herein and to avoid all potential hazards. By following the instructions contained herein, the reader willingly assumes all risks in connection with such instructions.

The publisher makes no representations or warranties of any kind, including but not limited to, the warranties of fitness for particular purpose or merchantability, nor are any such representations implied with respect to the material set forth herein, and the publisher takes no responsibility with respect to such material. The publisher shall not be liable for any special, consequential, or exemplary damages resulting, in whole or part, from the reader's use of, or reliance upon, this material.

Introduction . . . . **vii**

Effective Teaching Strategies . . . . **xi**

Module 1 | **Body Mechanics** **1**

General Information/Overview • 2
Audience Interaction for Transparency Master 1-2 • 2
Common Back Injuries • 3
Consequences of Back Injury • 3
Body Mechanics • 4
Structures Involved in Body Mechanics • 4
Ligaments and Muscles of the Back • 5
Facts about Back Pain • 5
Audience Interaction for Transparency Master 1-7 • 6
Elements of Body Mechanics • 6
Additional Audience Interaction for Transparency Master 1-7 • 7
Audience Interaction for Transparency Master 1-8 • 7
Principles of Body Mechanics • 8
Real-Life Scenario • 10
Demonstration: Body Alignment • 11
Group Activity • 12
Resource • 12
References • 13
Handouts and Transparency Masters • 14

Module 2 | **Safety** **25**

General Information/Overview • 26
Back Care • 27
Fire Safety • 28
Audience Interaction for Transparency Master 2-2 • 32
Fire Safety Questions and Answers • 32
Oxygen Safety • 33
Safety in the Home • 34
Audience Interaction for General Lecture Material • 34
Falls • 35
Crime Prevention • 36

Audience Interaction for Transparency Master 2-5 • 38
Safety in the Field • 40
Home-Visit Safety • 42
Fraud • 44
Audience Interaction for General Lecture Material • 45
Real-Life Scenario • 45
Demonstration: Proper Way to Stand • 46
Demonstration: Proper Way to Transfer a Client from
    Wheelchair to Chair • 46
Group Activity • 47
Resources • 47
References • 48
Handouts and Transparency Masters • 49

Module 3 — Abuse ... 61

Child Abuse • 62
General Information/Overview • 62
History • 62
Types of Maltreatment • 63
Causes of Child Abuse and Neglect • 67
Effects of Child Abuse and Neglect • 68
Reporting Child Abuse and Neglect • 69
Steps to Prevent Child Maltreatment • 69
Audience Interaction for General Lecture Material • 69

Domestic Violence • 70
General Information/Overview • 70
Types of Domestic Violence • 71
Characteristics of a Battered Woman • 72
Characteristics of the Abuser • 73
Factors Contributing to Abusive Behavior • 73
Signs of Domestic Abuse • 74
Reasons Battered Women Stay • 74
Preventing Domestic Violence • 75

Elder Abuse • 76
General Information/Overview • 76
History • 76
Categories of Elder Abuse • 77
Types of Elder Abuse • 77
Characteristics of Elder Abusers • 81
Factors Leading to Abuse • 81
Reporting Elder Abuse • 83
Preventing Elder Abuse • 83
Real-Life Scenario • 85
Group Activity • 86
Resources • 86
References • 87
Handouts and Transparency Masters • 88

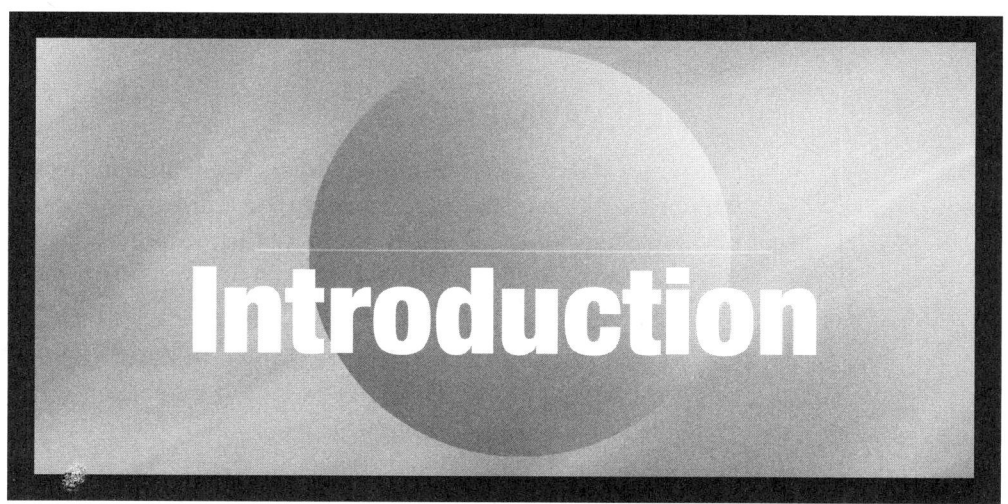

Community-based health care is needed in our society. The twenty-first century brings change to many aspects of our lives, including technology and medical breakthroughs. Despite the advancements, we are now facing more health care challenges than ever before. As health care reimbursement diminishes, many families are forced to care for their loved ones at home, with little or no training. Education is essential for successful health care in the home by family members or formal caregivers.

Home Care Aide Inservice Training Module: Safety is an all-inclusive set of inservices. Designed to allow the educator to present an inservice with little preparation time, each module includes PowerPoint® transparency masters and research materials for a one-hour presentation. This product presents a broad application for home care agencies and also provides valuable information for informal caregivers and support groups. The presenter should review the material before the inservice. Depending on the topic and the size of the audience, the instructional method may combine lecture, group discussion, demonstration, and group activities. Each module presents options for customizing the various instructional methods. Audience size, diversity, preferred learning style, and the setting for the presentation are important considerations when determining the optimal combination of methods. Using a combination of teaching strategies and tools results in a more effective presentation, which enhances learning and improves teaching-learning efficiency.

The use of visual aids is essential when using *Home Care Aide Inservice Training Module: Safety*. Visual aids increase information retention. Transparency masters are provided for each module to correspond to the Microsoft PowerPoint® slides, which are available on the free PowerPoint® CD packaged at the end of this book.

At the end of each module, instructional tools are included to summarize important concepts. Group activities, real-life scenarios including discussion questions and answers, and group demonstrations can be used to follow up the presentation. References and resources are also included with each module for further study.

NOTE: This book contains Modules 1–3 found in the complete package, *Home Care Aide: Inservice Training Modules* binder.

ALSO AVAILABLE:

Home Care Aide Inservice Module: Safety is one in a series of four separate inservice modules. Each module is made up of mini-modules that are designed for a one-hour inservice. All of the mini-modules include group activities, real-life scenarios with discussion questions and answers, transparency masters, and a free PowerPoint® CD. The other modules are:

Home Care Aide Inservice Module: Infection Control ISBN: 1-4018-9758-4
    Understanding Multidrug Resistant Bacteria
    Understanding Tuberculosis
    Understanding Hepatitis
    Understanding HIV and AIDS

Home Care Aide Inservice Module: Patient Care ISBN: 1-4018-9759-2
    Observation and Reporting
    Caring for the Skin
    Caring for the Cardiac Client
    Caring for the Client with Cerebrovascular Accident (CVA)
    Caring for the Client with Chronic Obstructive Pulmonary Disease (COPD)
    Caring for the Client with Diabetes
    Caring for the Client with Alzheimer's Disease
    Caring for the Client with Disabilities
    Caring for the Post-Operative Client
    Caring for the Aging Client

Home Care Aide Inservice Module: Supportive Measures ISBN: 1-4018-9760-6
    Healthy Eating
    Preventive Health Care
    Caring for the Dying Client

Complete Package!

Home Care Aide: Inservice Training Modules ISBN: 0-7668-3902-8
If you are looking for a complete package, we offer all four modules in one 3-ring binder with all the print materials found in the separate modules.
- Safety
- Infection Control
- Patient Care
- Supportive Measures

Additional Resources

The following products are perfect for training new home health aides or to complement your inservices.

- ***Basic Skills for Home Care Aides DVD Series*** (5-DVD Set)
  ISBN: 1-4018-3182-6
  Perfect to complement your inservice training, this 5-DVD series presents the procedures required by OBRA for home care aides in an easy-to-follow, step-by-step format. By allowing learners to observe the skills from start to

finish, they will have a better understanding of everything they need to know for each skill, including all necessary equipment. By concentrating on the core skills required to pass the national home care certification exam, learners will be able to view all the steps needed to complete each skill on which they will be tested.

Each DVD is also available individually.

DVD 1 ISBN: 1-4018-3183-4
    Segment 1: Orientation to Home Health Care and Communication
    Segment 2: Infection Control and Safety

DVD 2 ISBN: 1-4018-03184-2
    Segment 3: Body Mechanics
    Segment 4: Rehabilitation Skills

DVD 3 ISBN: 1-4018-3186-9
    Segment 5: Personal Hygiene and Grooming
    Segment 6: Personal Care

DVD 4 ISBN: 1-4018-3187-7
    Segment 7: Nutrition and Fluid Balance
    Segment 8: Elimination

DVD 5 ISBN: 1-4018-3188-5
    Segment 9: Vital Signs, Pain, and Medication
    Segment 10: Special Treatments and Caring for the Dying

- *Homemaker/Home Health Aide: On the Job Companion*
ISBN: 1-4018-3145-1
This handbook is designed as a reference to provide essential information to assist in caring for clients in the home, assisted living arrangements, and group homes. It is also a useful tool in helping the learner transition from the classroom setting to practice.

- *Homemaker/Home Health Aide Exam Review*
ISBN: 1-4018-3143-5
This product was written to help prepare the learner for the national home care aide written certification exam. The book is organized into three sections based on the National Home Care Association's *A Model Curriculum and Teaching Guide for Instruction of the Homemaker-Home Health Aide.* It contains 24 chapters with over 1,500 questions with answers and rationales as to why answers are correct or incorrect.

- *Homemaker/Home Health Aide, 5e* by Audree Spatz and Suzann
  Balduzzi
ISBN: 1-4018-3139-7
A comprehensive text designed for use in initial training programs for home health aides, and as a reference in required continuing education courses. The practical applications of procedures required by OBRA are included in each unit. The book is designed to train individuals entering the field for the first time, and practicing home health aides to be caring, dedicated, and skilled paraprofessionals. The role of the home health aide as a valuable member of the health care team is emphasized throughout the book. A *free* study CD-ROM that reinforces concepts in the book in a fun game format is packaged with each book.

To enhance the learning and teaching experience of this product, we have developed:

- *Workbook to Accompany Homemaker/Home Health Aide, 5e*
  ISBN: 1-4018-3142-7
  This workbook is designed to enhance your instruction. Each chapter of the workbook is correlated to a unit in the textbook and includes learning objectives, terms to define, application exercises, crossword puzzles, and quizzes to reinforce the core concepts found in the text.

For the Instructor:

- *Instructor's Manual to Accompany Homemaker/Home Health Aide, 5e*
  ISBN: 1-4018-3140-0
  This includes teaching tips and strategies, course syllabus, unit lesson plans, class activities, additional review questions, case studies with questions, answers to textbook review questions and case studies, and answers to the review questions in the workbook.

- *Computerized Testbank to Accompany Homemaker/Home Health Aide, 5e*
  ISBN: 1-4018-3141-9
  This CD-ROM includes over 1,300 questions and answers organized according to the 26 units in the textbook. The testbank assists you in creating personalized unit tests.

ACKNOWLEDGMENTS

The authors and Delmar Learning wish to thank the following reviewers for their review of the manuscript:

Laura J. Ninger, ELS
Medical Editing and Writing
Rutherford, NJ

Linda Sutterley, RN, BSN
Home Health Generalist
VNA Home Care of Mercer County
Trenton, NJ

Joann B. Tharrington, RN
Nurse Aide Instructor/Coordinator
Edgecombe Community College
Rocky Mount, NC

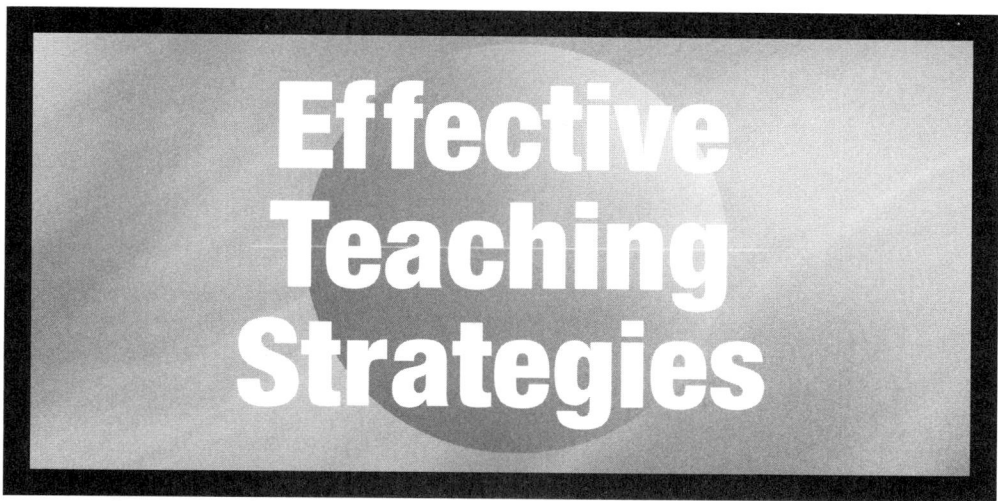

A successful presentation includes more than just accurate research material. Success entails the combination of both the material and the ability to keep the audience interested in the topic.

Be Enthusiastic

Present the information so that the audience becomes excited about the subject. Talk to everyone in the group by maintaining eye contact and changing positions and direction. Use body language to emphasize important issues.

Use Humor

The use of humor in any situation reduces anxiety and helps maintain the learners' attention. However, joke telling is not a requirement. Be yourself. Do not try too hard to be funny or something you are not.

Take Risks

The only way to know if a new teaching method is going to work is to try it. Do not get discouraged if the audience does not respond at first. Try a new approach and see what happens. Every audience is unique.

Incorporate Real-Life Examples

Some of the inservice material is technical. The learner wants to know, "Why is this important to me?" Throughout the presentation, mention real-life examples so that the learner will value the information provided.

Be Flexible

Depending on the topic and the audience, the instructional method may need to change. Although the teacher may prefer a specific style, such as group discussion, certain topics and learners may require a different method. Assess the atmosphere and teach accordingly.

Initiate Thought-Provoking Activities

The audience needs to take the information and incorporate it into their everyday thinking. The teacher needs to challenge the audience by having them develop solutions to problems. Propose questions, brainstorming, or testing to promote problem-solving skills.

Be Prepared

If you are not prepared for the presentation, the class will not value the information. You do not have to be an expert on every subject, but you do have to review the information presented. Be prepared to refer audiences to sources where they can find information, such as organizations, books, and articles. Do not give false information.

Get Feedback

The teacher and the learner need to seek information about the quality of their performance. Feedback should be encouraged during and at the end of each presentation. It can be obtained from verbal and nonverbal responses. The instructor should observe for nonverbal clues, such as lack of eye contact from the audience and restlessness. Teaching strategies may need to be changed accordingly. The teacher may ask questions such as, "Is this clear?" or "Did I answer your question?"

Reinforce Important Items

During a presentation, always reinforce the key points of the session. Emphasize the terms you want the learner to remember. Statements such as, "again we see," "as mentioned before," or "remember" are reminders to the audience.

Summarize Key Points

At the end of any teaching session, summarize the important points. This will reinforce the teaching-learning process and provide feedback as to the progress made.

Tips for Using Transparencies and Slides

Visual aids increase the audience's retention of the material. Combining what we hear with what we see is an effective teaching approach. Visual aids should enhance the presentation and not detract from it. The teacher should do the following:

- Turn off the projector when not in use. The fan noise can be distracting.
- Expand on the information or provide complete handouts.
- Display one point at a time by masking the rest with a piece of paper. The learner can concentrate on that item.
- The screen should be large enough for the audience to read the information.
- Read from the screen that the audience sees, not from your notes.

Source: Bastable, S. B. (1997). *Nurse as educator, principles of teaching and learning.* London: Jones and Bartlett.

Module 1
Body Mechanics

GOAL
To understand the principles of body mechanics and how they apply to everyday life

OBJECTIVES
After completion of the presentation, students will be able to:
- Define the term *body mechanics*.
- Describe the importance of proper body mechanics.
- Demonstrate the center of gravity using a wide base.
- Identify at least eight principles of body mechanics.
- Describe how to lift a heavy object from the floor using proper body mechanics.

2 • SAFETY

Lecture Material for Transparency Master 1-1

● GENERAL INFORMATION/OVERVIEW

Every year health care workers gather and review the fundamentals of body mechanics, yet back injuries still occur.

- Back injuries account for a majority of worker's compensation cases and loss of work.
- Decreased productivity and loss of work make a back injury very expensive for the employer.
- Body mechanics is more than dollars and cents. The audience must understand that the responsibility for proper care of the back lies with them, because it affects their lives.
- Just as a bad back can interfere with everyday activities, a fit back can assist you in leading an active, healthy life.
- A bad back is not inevitable, but is affected by lifestyle and habits (such as excess weight, smoking, and lack of exercise). Poor posture, twisting movements, and improper lifting can increase the risk of injuries.
- If you experience a backache, do not ignore it! Notify the agency's supervisor and contact your physician. Reevaluate your performance of the task that caused the injury.

Lecture Material for Transparency Master 1-2

Body mechanics is the coordinated use of body parts to produce motion and maintain balance. Body mechanics includes:

- The way we move, how we stand, and how we sit
- Our ability to perform all of our activities of daily living

● AUDIENCE INTERACTION FOR TRANSPARENCY MASTER 1-2

Ask the audience to name some possible problems associated with poor or improper use of body mechanics. You may want to lead the audience with possible scenarios, such as the following:

- What happens when you lift something that may be too heavy?
- How do you feel after you do the laundry?
- How do you feel after sitting in the movie theater or an inservice meeting?
- What happens after you lift a heavy client?
- Are you able to care for others?

Lecture Material for Transparency Master 1-3

Improper use of body mechanics can lead to multiple injuries. Prolonged activities and fatigue can also contribute to these impairments.

COMMON BACK INJURIES

- Low-back sprains and strains are the most common causes of back pain. The pain usually occurs after a sudden forceful movement, causing injuries to a ligament.
- Some injuries involve the intervertebral disks. These occur when there is a weakening in the disk, causing compression of the spaces between the vertebrae. Protruding disk, herniated disk, or slipped disk are terms used to describe such injuries.
- Facet-joint osteoarthritis is a degenerative arthritis of the spine. The arthritic changes cause pain and stiffness in the back, which can be exacerbated by improper body mechanics.

CONSEQUENCES OF BACK INJURY

Loss of Work

- According to the National Council on Compensation Insurance, 25% of worker's compensation claims are attributed to back injuries.
- An average of 555 million days of work are lost per year because of back pain and injuries.

Chronic Back Pain

- It is easier to prevent a back injury than to eliminate the pain of an injury.
- It is difficult to identify the cause of back pain because it can originate in the soft tissue, bones, disks, or nerves.
- No magic remedy or foolproof treatment plan exists for back pain. It can be difficult to treat.
- Back exercises can strengthen muscles and reduce pain.

Inability to Care for Others

- Injured, weak, or tense muscles and ligaments cause pain and limit the ability to care for others.
- Injury can cause financial hardship if the client is unable to work.
- If a caregiver is unable to care for a family member, the caregiver will have the additional burden of finding a replacement or assistance.

● BODY MECHANICS

Everyone should apply the principles of body mechanics at all times.

- Proper body mechanics are necessary in all activities, from elevating a client's extremity to cooking, cleaning, and doing laundry.
- Using these principles can keep the expenditure of energy to a minimum when lifting, moving, or carrying a heavy object.
- The principles of body mechanics should be taught from a young age.

Lecture Material for Transparency Master 1-4

The instructor can teach all the necessary information about proper body mechanics, but if these principles are not followed, back pain may occur.

- As caregivers, we must first take care of ourselves. Without the home care aide (HCA) or caregiver, the client will not get the needed help. This is important to remember.
- Using the principles of body mechanics is another way to "take care of you."

Lecture Material for Transparency Master 1-5

This portion will review the basic elements of the human body as they relate to body mechanics.

● STRUCTURES INVOLVED IN BODY MECHANICS

Spinal Cord

- The spinal cord enables movement.
- When properly aligned, the spine curves gently inward at the neck and lower back and outward in the rib area.
- This "S" shape keeps the head, chest, and pelvis centered, balancing the weight of the body.

Intervertebral Disks

- Disks are the pads of soft tissue between the 26 vertebrae.
- This padding allows the bony spine to twist and move easily.

Vertebrae

- Vertebrae are the bones of the spine.
- The spinal cord and nerves run through the vertebrae.
- Vertebrae support the back and protect the spinal cord.

Lecture Material for Transparency Master 1-6

LIGAMENTS AND MUSCLES OF THE BACK

- Hip and leg muscles, as well as back muscles, are involved when lifting a heavy weight.
- Back muscles are used for lighter work.
- The superficial back muscles do not move the trunk of the body.
- The smaller, deeper muscles are responsible for movement of the body trunk.
- Strong abdominal muscles will aid the lower back muscles.
- The back muscles must be strong to sustain whatever effort is put forth. Otherwise, the ligaments alone may have to withstand the force, which can cause injury.
- Hamstrings and quadriceps are the larger leg muscles, and should be used to lift a heavy object, rather than the smaller ones of the back.

FACTS ABOUT BACK PAIN

- Any activity, if performed incorrectly and repetitively, can weaken the back.
- Back pain can last from a few days to a few weeks, and the symptoms can last a lifetime.
- Backs do not just "give out." Injury is related to an accumulation of weakness, including wear and tear on untoned muscles, poor posture, obesity, and stress.
- Back pain is a protective response of the body. When a task puts too much pressure on a muscle, an involuntary muscle contraction or spasm can occur.
- Stress can contribute to injury because stress causes a chronic shortening and tightening of muscles, which can trigger a spasm. This spasm decreases the damage indirectly by causing the individual to stop the activity.
- With age, the cushioning disks separating the vertebrae of the back lose their elasticity and moisture, and then shrink, possibly causing muscle pain and herniation of the disk.
- The spasm may be relieved by lying down, which reduces stress on the back and allows the inflamed tissue to repair itself.
- Most injuries occur to the lower back because this is the largest curve in the spine and supports the most weight.

6 ● SAFETY

Lecture Material for Transparency Master 1-7

● AUDIENCE INTERACTION FOR TRANSPARENCY MASTER 1-7

Ask the audience to look at how everyone is sitting in the chairs. (Get feedback from them.)

- Poor posture places increased stress on the spine.
- When correctly aligned, the spine curves inward at the neck and lower back and outward in the rib area. Look at how the back is curved now.
- Rounded shoulders, a slumped position, or an excessive arch causes a weight imbalance that adds strain to the back. Over time, this causes narrowing between the vertebrae, leading to a condition called a *bulging disk*.
- Evaluate your posture in the mirror when sitting or standing to see if you maintain the "S" curve.
- Regular exercise, including cardiovascular exercise and stretching for flexibility, is essential for back strength.
- When standing, the vertebrae tend to compress on themselves, increasing the lower arch. Use a footstool and rest one leg on it to flatten the spinal curve when standing for a long period.

● ELEMENTS OF BODY MECHANICS

Center of Gravity

- Explain how each line divides the body into planes. The point where the lines intersect is the *center of gravity*.
- Stability is increased when the base of support is broad and the center of gravity is low. The broader the base, the greater the stability.
- The skeletal system is designed so an imaginary line could be dropped from the top of the head to the bottom of the feet.
- The body is well balanced and has several natural curves in the neck and upper back, as well as the lower back and tailbone ("S" shape).
- The center of gravity will differ in individuals according to their build, and will vary with every change in body posture.

Balance

- When everything is aligned, the body maintains a *balance*.
- Improper lifting or bending can cause changes in body alignment, leading to falls or injuries.

Posture

- *Posture* is the position and alignment of masses of the human body.
- The body is designed like an architectural structure and is subject to the laws of gravity.
- The body needs to be continually realigned to allow proper function.
- When the body is not properly aligned, there is a chance of muscle, back, and spinal injury; improper alignment can even affect the functions of vital organs.

- Slouching forward restricts the movement of the lungs.
- Poor body alignment in a chair can make you sluggish and slow down blood supply to the brain.

ADDITIONAL AUDIENCE INTERACTION FOR TRANSPARENCY MASTER 1-7

Have you ever felt that you were going to lose your balance, but did not fall? This occurs because you regained or maintained the center of gravity.

Lecture Material for Transparency Master 1-8

We can create a wide base with different techniques.

1. Spread your feet about hip-length apart. Have your feet and knees face in the same direction.
2. Place one foot in front of you and the other foot behind you. (This is called the *athletic stance.*)

Demonstrate both techniques for the audience, illustrating how the positions maintain balance.

- By using proper body mechanics, you can maintain the center of gravity and the alignment of the back.
- Bring heavy items close to you before lifting. This prevents your body from moving out of alignment while maintaining your center of gravity though the base of support. Bring the client closer to you when transferring him.

What are the principles of body mechanics?

- The principles of body mechanics are based on the theories of physics.
- Simple everyday activities are made easier because of the properties of motion and force.
- When lifting a heavy object, we tend to bring the object close to the body because it is easier to handle. The fact is that we are bringing the object into our center of gravity, or into the plane in which we move.
- We push heavy boxes rather than pull them because it is easier, again because of the forces of gravity and friction.

AUDIENCE INTERACTION FOR TRANSPARENCY MASTER 1-8

What else can proper body mechanics do?

- By using proper body mechanics in our everyday activities, we can do less work.
- Proper alignment of body parts and the correct application of scientific principles in lifting and carrying heavy objects help to conserve energy.

Lecture Material for Handout 1-3

Incorporating the principles of body mechanics into our daily routines helps prevent back pain. The abdominal (stomach) muscles are the supporting muscles of the back and must be strengthened and stretched. The proper way to bend and move must be relearned to decrease muscle strain on the back. Proper exercising can increase the strength of muscles.

● PRINCIPLES OF BODY MECHANICS

Always Have a Stable Base of Support and Maintain the Center of Gravity

- The broader the base, the greater the stability.
- When everything is aligned, the body maintains a proper balance.
- Stability is increased when the base of support is broad and the center of gravity is low.

Get Close to the Load That You Are Lifting

- Bring the work closer to you.
- Bring the object to your center of gravity; if you do not, the weight will pull you out of alignment and you may lose your balance.
- When giving a bed bath, have the client move closer to you.
- Bring the grocery bags closer to you when carrying them.

Use the Larger Muscles or Muscle Groups

- If you reach with your arm to sit a client up in bed, you are using just the biceps muscle.
- If you bend your elbow under a client's underarm and sit him or her up, you are using the muscles in the arm, shoulder, and back.
- Use the larger leg muscles to bend rather than the smaller and weaker muscles of the back.

Use Proper Posture

- Poor posture creates undue pressure on the muscles, ligaments, and vertebrae.
- Proper posture creates good body alignment.
- Good body alignment encourages the correct function of all body systems.

If You Think It Is Too Heavy to Lift Alone, Get Help

- Do not do anything that will cause injury to yourself or others.
- Use common sense.

Use Coordinated Movements

- Jerky movements cause undue strain on the joints.
- Explain what you are doing to your partner or to the client.
- Set up a plan. For example, "On the count of three, you are going to stand. . . .1, 2, 3, stand."

Plan the Move

- Be prepared.
  - Is there a clear passage to where the object is being moved?
  - Before a transfer, is the client's wheelchair positioned properly?
  - Are there objects on the floor?
  - Is there enough light in the room where you are going?
- Explain the procedure to the client.

Better to Push, Pull, or Roll an Object Than to Lift and Carry It

- Lifting requires moving the weight of the object against the pull of gravity.
- Pushing or pulling uses less energy than lifting.
- Try to push, pull, or roll rather than lift.

Use Your Leg Muscles to Lift an Object, Not Your Arms or Back

- Your leg muscles are the largest muscle groups in the body.
- Use your arms to anchor the object you are lifting.
- Maintain the natural curve in your back.

Work With the Direction of Your Efforts, Not Against Them

- Your feet should always point toward the direction of the work; this will avoid a twisting motion in the knees.
- When assisting a client to sit up in bed (you can demonstrate this method):
  - Point your feet toward the client.
  - Maintain the wide base and center of gravity.
  - Use your upper arm and shoulder muscles to help the client sit up.

Bring the Work to a Comfortable Position

- If there is a hospital bed, raise it to a level at which you are not bending.
- Lower yourself to the level of the work so you are not bending. For example, sit on a chair when giving a bed bath.

- Bring the client closer to the side of the bed where you are working.
- Avoid kneeling because it can cause pressure and pain to the knee area and the floor may not be safe (e.g., nails, debris). Use a kneeling pad if there is no other choice.

Avoid Twisting Motions

- Twisting causes strain on the back.
- The strain can irritate the nerves, causing spasms.

Reinforce to the audience the importance of both the principles of body mechanics and the need to maintain a healthy back.

Instructor's version with answers for Handout 1-2

● REAL-LIFE SCENARIO

A nurse was giving a lecture on body mechanics and explained how in nursing school, she had a class on this topic. The instructor demonstrated and explained the various techniques for transferring and lifting clients. The nurse stated that she understood the lesson, but not its importance. Not even a week later, while transferring a client from a bed to a chair, she injured her back. She was in bed for a week and continues to have back problems today. She realizes now that the lesson on the proper use of body mechanics was for her safety: not for a grade, not for an inservice credit, but for her own well-being.

Question 1. What is proper body mechanics?

Answer: Body mechanics is the coordinated use of body parts to produce motion and maintain balance.

Question 2. Why do you think she injured her back?

Answer: The HCA injured her back by not using the principles of body mechanics. Review handout for principles of body mechanics.

Question 3. Why are proper body mechanics so important to you?

Answer: Proper body mechanics are important to avoid injury, chronic back pain, loss of work, and limitation of activities.

Question 4. Describe your concerns about using the principles of body mechanics.

Answer: Possible concerns for students can involve the realities of home care. The HCA is alone in the home and does not have the luxury of asking someone to assist with transfers. The needed equipment may not be available to the HCA. The client may be uncooperative and resist the HCA. All concerns should be discussed with the supervisor.

DEMONSTRATION

BODY ALIGNMENT

Proper body alignment allows the muscles and joints to function correctly. When alignment is maintained, the muscles divide the work, conserving energy and preventing fatigue. For proper alignment, the body is straight, but not tense.

Proper Way to Stand

1. The feet face forward in the same direction as the knees.
2. The legs are straight, but not tense.
3. The spine is long. Do not slouch.
4. The curves of the spinal column are within normal limits (the "S" shape is maintained).
5. The head is upright.

Positioning a Client in Bed

When positioning a client in bed, the alignment of his body is the same as in a proper standing posture. The curves of the spine are maintained, the head is supported in line with the midline of the trunk, and rotation of the spine is avoided. (The neck, shoulders, and hips are all in alignment. The spinal cord is straight.) This alignment is maintained in all positions: back (supine), side lying, or stomach (prone). Support injured parts of the body. The rest should be left free to move. This will help the blood to circulate.

Moving a Client

A typical task is moving a client from the center to the side of the bed. If the client can assist, have him or her do as much as possible.

1. Explain the procedure to the client.
2. Stand on the side of the bed where you want the client to lie.
3. Place the client's arms across the chest.
4. Maintain a wide base.
5. Move the client's legs toward you.
6. Place your hands under each hip of the client and gently move the hips toward you. The hips may move only an inch or so at a time.
7. Place your hands under each shoulder of the client and gently move the upper torso toward you. The torso may move only an inch or so at a time.
8. Continue the above three steps until the client is at the determined site.
9. Assess the client for proper body alignment and position.

Vacuuming

1. Place one foot in front of the other foot.
2. Move back and forth by shifting the weight from foot to foot (not just moving the arm back and forth).
3. Bend from the hips to lower the torso.

GROUP ACTIVITY

For a small group:

Have everyone demonstrate picking up a box or laundry basket, and critique their form using comments from the class.

For a large group:

Select volunteers from the audience and have them demonstrate picking up a box or laundry basket. Critique their form using comments from the audience.

*Omit any persons who have a history of back problems from performing the demonstration.

Explain the proper way to lift a laundry basket from the floor.

1. Keep both feet flat on the floor.
2. Spread the legs hip-width apart (about 10–12") for a broad base of support. If using the athletic stance, one foot should be in front of the other.
3. Stand as close to the laundry basket as possible.
4. Face the laundry basket (no twisting).
5. Bend the knees.
6. Hold the basket and lift by straightening the knees. The lifting is done by the largest and strongest muscles of the legs (quadriceps femoris).
7. Maintain the natural "S" curve of the back.
8. Move the feet or pivot to place the basket on the counter. (Do not twist the back.)

 RESOURCE

Guide for proper body mechanics:
http://www.rehabnet.com

REFERENCES

Fishman, L., & Ardman, C. (1997). *Back talk: How to diagnose & cure low back pain and sciatica.* London: W.W. Norton & Co.

Lagerwerff, E. (1977). *Mensendieck; Your posture and your pains.* New York: Anchor/Doubleday.

Maharan, L. (1998). *A healthy back: A sport medicine doctor's back-care program for everybody.* New York: Henry Holt.

Rhodes, M. (1996, January). Back in balance. *Women's Sports & Fitness, 18,* 44–49.

Seedor, M. (1997). *Body mechanics and patient positioning: A program unit for nurses.* New York: Teachers College Press.

Time-Life Books. (1988). *The fit back, prevention and recovery.* Alexandria, VA: Time-Life.

YMCA of the USA with Patricia Sammann. (1994). *YMCA health back book.* Champaign, IL: Human Kinetics Publishers.

Name _____ Date _____

Program/Course _____ Instructor's Name _____

BODY MECHANICS
Pre/Post Test

1. What is the major cause of absenteeism in the workplace?
    a. the flu
    b. back injuries
    c. falls
    d. respiratory conditions

2. *Body mechanics* is defined as:
    a. the way in which our body works.
    b. the coordinated use of body parts to produce motion and maintain balance.
    c. a framework in which illness is studied in relation to functional systems of the body.
    d. the whole structure of an individual with all the organs.

3. The improper use of body mechanics can lead to:
    a. back pain.
    b. loss of work.
    c. limited ability to care for others.
    d. all of the above.

4. Stability is increased when the base of support is broad and the center of gravity is low. This occurs when we:
    a. maintain a wide base of support.
    b. slouch.
    c. lose our balance and fall.
    d. none of the above.

5. Which statement is *not* part of the principles of body mechanics?
    a. Always have a stable base of support.
    b. Maintain the center of gravity.
    c. If you think it is too heavy to lift alone, get help.
    d. Do not bend your knees.

Handout **1-1**

Name _____ Date _____

Program/Course _____ Instructor's Name _____

REAL-LIFE SCENARIO

A nurse was giving a lecture on body mechanics and explained how in nursing school, she had a class on this topic. The instructor demonstrated and explained the various techniques for transferring and lifting clients. The nurse stated she understood the lesson, but not its importance. Not even a week later, while transferring a client from a bed to a chair, she injured her back. She was in bed for a week and continues to have back problems today. She realizes now the lesson on the proper use of body mechanics was for her safety: not for a grade, not for an inservice credit, but for her own well-being.

Question 1. What is proper body mechanics?

Question 2. Why do you think she injured her back?

Question 3. Why are proper body mechanics so important to you?

Question 4. Describe your concerns about using the principles of body mechanics.

Handout **1-2**

Copyright © 2005 by Delmar Learning, a division of Thomson Learning, Inc.

PRINCIPLES OF BODY MECHANICS

* Always have a stable base of support.
* Maintain the center of gravity.
* Get close to the load that is being lifted.
* Use the larger muscles or muscle groups.
* Use proper posture.
* If you think it is too heavy to lift alone, *get help.*
* Use coordinated movements.
* Plan the move.
* It is better to push, pull, or roll an object than to lift and carry it.
* Use your leg muscles to lift an object, not your arm or back muscles.
* Work with the direction of your efforts, not against them.
* Bring your work to a comfortable position.
* Avoid twisting motions.

BODY MECHANICS

Body mechanics is the coordinated use of body parts to produce motion and maintain balance.

Improper use of body mechanics can lead to:
- **Injuries**
- **Loss of work**
- **Chronic back pain**
- **Inability to care for others**

The responsibility lies with you.

Structures involved in body mechanics

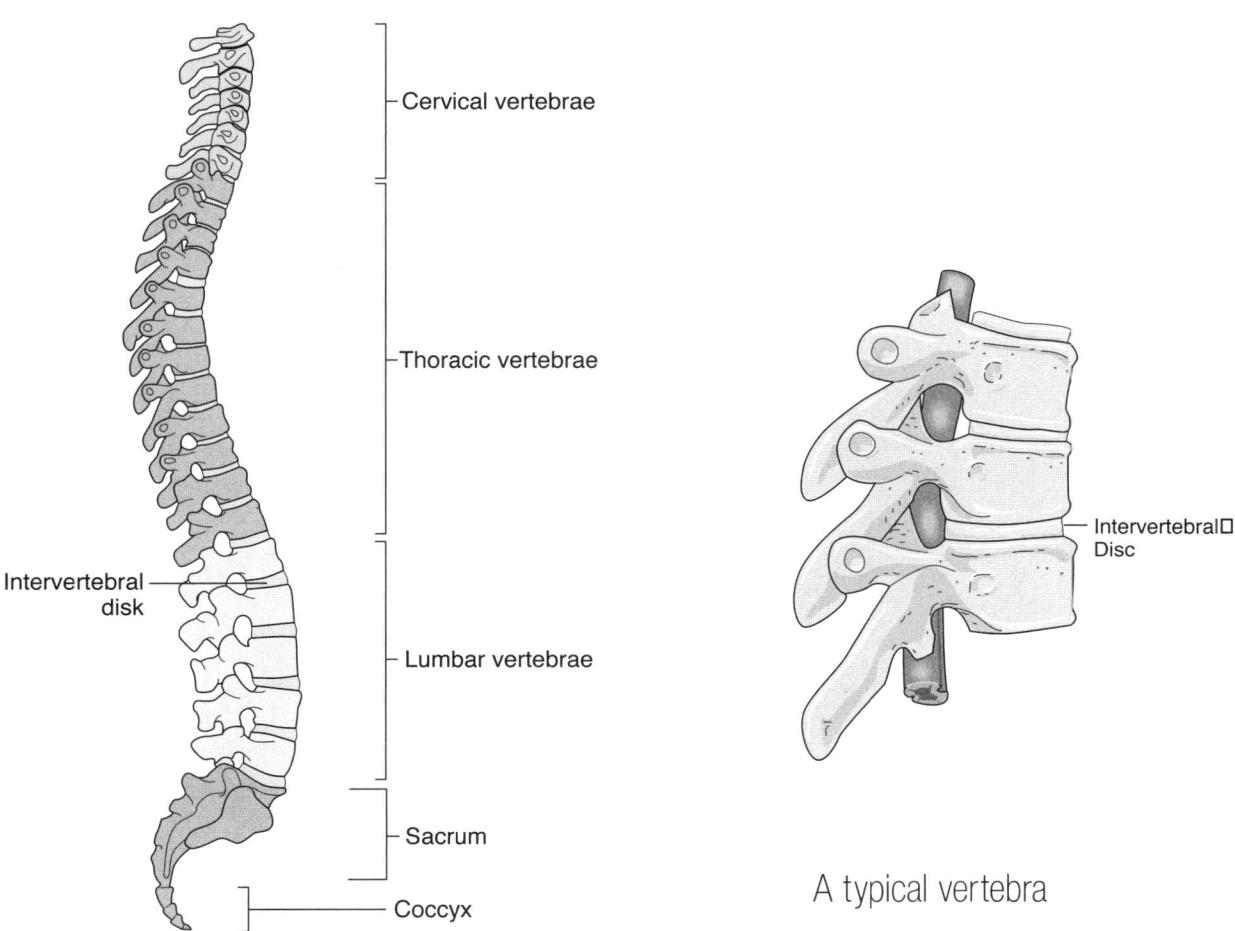

Side view of the spinal cord

A typical vertebra

Muscles of the back

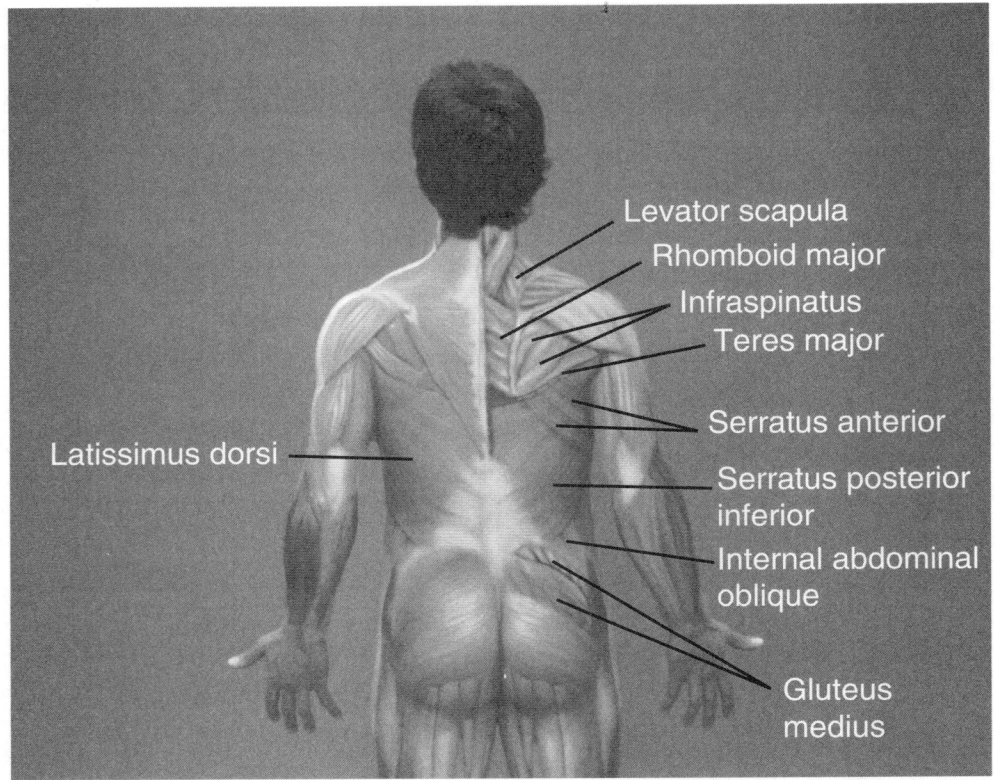

Center of gravity

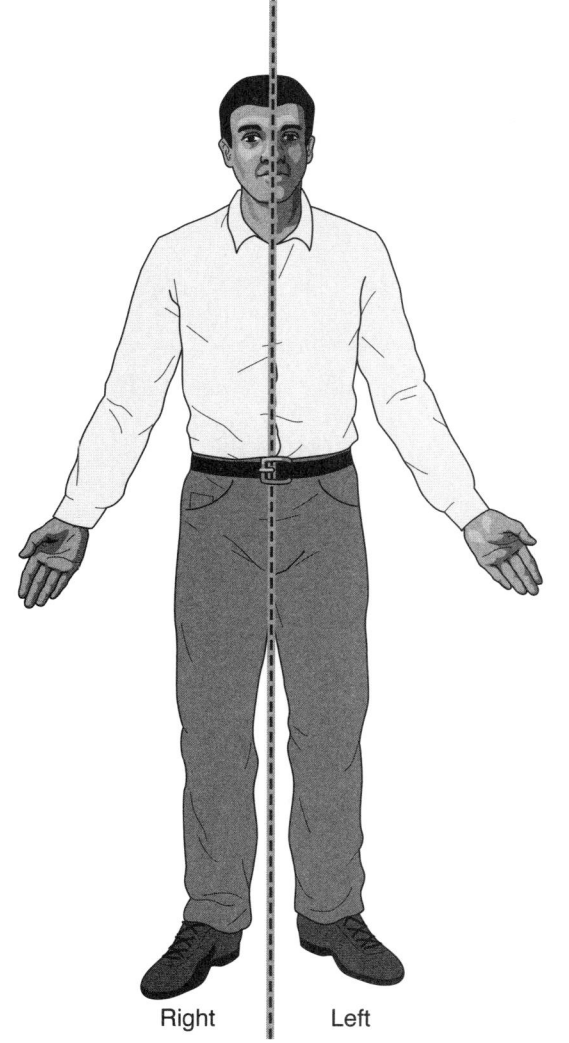

Right | Left

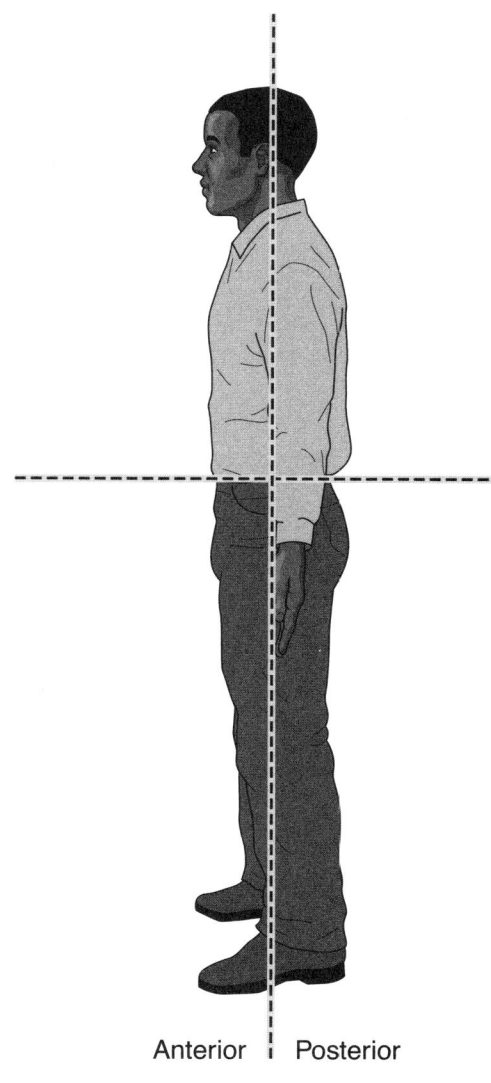

Anterior | Posterior

Transparency Master **1-7**

Body mechanics

Narrow base of support

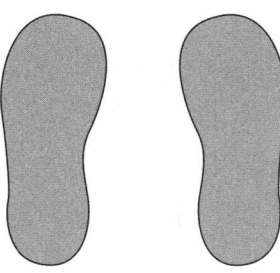

Wide base of support

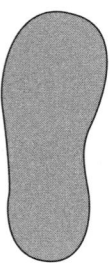 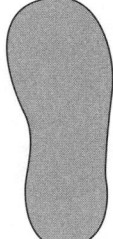

Module 2
Safety

GOAL
To establish guidelines to ensure client and employee safety

OBJECTIVES
After completion of the presentation, students will be able to:

- Demonstrate the proper way to transfer a client from a wheelchair to a chair while using proper body mechanics.
- Explain what is meant by E.D.I.T.H.
- Describe what actions to take in the event of a fire.
- List four preventive measures to reduce falls in the home.
- Define *workplace violence*.
- List six home-visit safety guidelines.

26 • SAFETY

Lecture Material for Transparency Master 2-1

● GENERAL INFORMATION/OVERVIEW

When caring for the frail and elderly, safety issues become even more important because clients may not be capable of protecting themselves. Safety is everyone's responsibility. Home care aides (HCAs) are responsible for the safety of both the client and themselves.

- Always be aware of your surroundings; this can help prevent accidents.
- Always read the labels or instructions before using a new product (e.g., cleaning items, appliances).
- Do not use any equipment (e.g., Hoyer lift) on a client if the supervisor has not instructed you to do so.

The elderly client may have sensory loss, leading to the following:
- Decreased sense of smell, which may put them at risk for not smelling a fire or gas leak
- Hearing loss, which may prevent them from hearing alarms or sirens
- Visual changes, including difficulty in adapting from dark to light puts them at risk for falls, especially when getting up during the night.

The elderly may have delayed reaction time, which increases the risk of accidents.
- Reduction in fine motor skills can increase the risk of burns and lacerations (cuts), especially while cooking.
- Reduction in gross motor skills can cause an unsteady gate, which increases the risk of:
  - falls in the bathroom.
  - falls on the stairs.
  - falls during transfers.
- Evacuation from the home may be difficult if the client is homebound and unable to leave on her own.

Because of the following medical problems, some clients may be confused and unable to comprehend possible dangers.
- Clients with Alzheimer's disease
- Clients with altered mental status from stroke or brain injury
- Medicated clients

Most important, use common sense.
- Do not use a chair as a ladder.
- Many accidents occur because the HCA is trying to please the client or the family.
- The safety of the client always comes first; there are no exceptions.

- If you were not instructed on how to transfer the client using the Hoyer lift, do not transfer the client even if the client or client's family asks. Call the supervisor.
- Gut feelings and intuition are an important part of our safety defenses. If the voice inside tells you not to walk down that street, do not walk down that street.
- "When in doubt, do without!" If you are unsure whether to do something, wait for additional instructions.
- Notify the supervisor immediately when a safety concern arises.
- Notify the supervisor immediately if you or your client is injured.

(Insert your agency's policy for reporting injuries of HCAs and clients here.)

General Lecture Material — No Transparency Master

The following information is repeated in this module to satisfy state and federal requirements. Please check with your state for additional requirements for safety inservice.

BACK CARE

See Module 1 in this book for more information and overheads.

Back Injuries

Back injuries account for approximately one-half of all reported injuries and illnesses in the health care industry. Following the principles of body mechanics can reduce the HCA's risk of injury.

- Use proper body mechanics to maintain the center of gravity and alignment of the back and body.
- Bring heavy items close to you. This prevents your body from moving out of alignment, while maintaining your center of gravity through the base of support.
- Bring the client closer to you when transferring him or her.
- Remember that when maintaining the center of gravity, the body stays aligned, preventing back injuries.

Body Alignment

- Proper body alignment allows the muscles and joints to function correctly.
- When alignment is maintained, the muscles divide the work, conserving energy and preventing fatigue.

Preventing Back Pain

- The abdominal (stomach) muscles are the supporting muscles for the back and must be strengthened and stretched.
- The proper ways to bend and move must be learned; these techniques will decrease muscle strain on the back.
- Maintain a wide base.

Principles of Body Mechanics

Review Handout 1-3 on the principles of body mechanics located in Module 1 of this book.

- Always have a stable base of support.
- Spread your feet about hip-length apart. Have your feet and knees face in the same direction.
- Place one foot in front of you and the other foot behind you (the athletic stance).
- Always maintain the center of gravity.
- Get close to the load you are about to lift.
- Always use proper posture.
- If you think the load is too heavy to lift alone, get help.
- Always use coordinated movements.
- Plan your move.
- It is better to push, pull, or roll the object than to lift and carry it.
- Use your leg muscles to lift the object rather than your arm or back muscles.
- Work with the direction of your effort, not against it.
- Bring your work to a comfortable position.
- Avoid any twisting motions.

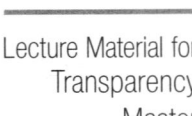

Lecture Material for Transparency Master 2-2

FIRE SAFETY

Fire Facts

Fire is the third leading cause of accidental deaths in homes. Most fires occur in the kitchen.

- Cooking is the leading cause of fires, usually because of leaving cooking unattended.
- The leading cause of fire deaths is smoking. The second leading cause of fires and fire deaths is faulty heating systems.
- The risk of fire deaths among seniors and children under the age of five is double that of the average population.
- Working smoke detectors and knowledge of the evacuation route increase the chances of survival.

Tips on Preventing Fires

- Store flammable items (e.g., aerosol cans) away from heat.
- Do not use items with frayed electrical wiring.
- Do not overload electrical outlets.
- Dispose of items properly (e.g., paints, stains, cigarettes).
- Do not leave cooking unattended.

- Turn handles of pots inward on the stove so they do not hang over the flames or get bumped by a passerby.
- Perform routine maintenance of home heating systems.
- Post emergency numbers by the telephone.
- Keep matches away from children.

Elements Needed for Fire

The three elements needed to start a fire are:
1. Fuel (something flammable).
2. Heat (something to start the flame).
3. Oxygen (the fire itself needs oxygen, or air).

Putting Out a Fire

By removing one of the necessary elements, you can prevent or stop a fire. To put out flames from a grease fire:
- Reduce the oxygen by smothering the flames with salt or with the lid of a pan.
- If clothing catches on fire when cooking:
  1. Remove the clothing and smother the flame by stamping it out (removing the oxygen).
  2. Pour water on it (reducing the flame).
  3. If you cannot remove the clothing, drop and roll on the floor, smothering the flames (removing the oxygen).

Have a Fire Plan

Having a fire exit plan is necessary to ensure a way out if a fire occurs. During a crisis, it is easy to become overwhelmed and panic.

Practice Exit Drills In The Home (E.D.I.T.H.).
1. Create an escape plan.
   - Draw a floor plan of your home.
   - Determine two ways to exit each room of the home. Stress the importance of being prepared.
   - Check windows and doors to determine whether there is easy access to the outside.
   - Use escape ladders or fire escapes for a multi-story home.
   - Security bars on the windows should have quick releases, and everyone should be instructed on how to use them.
2. Review the plan with members of the home.
   - Make sure everyone in the home is aware of escape routes.
   - Avoid clutter in hallways or walk areas to maintain a clear path for escape.

- Sleep with the doors closed. In the event of a fire, this reduces the heat and smoke in the room, which allows more time to evacuate.
- Check smoke detectors. They must be working to save lives. Remember that smoke detectors should be on each level in the home, in each bedroom, and outside of the sleeping areas.
- Periodically clean the dust out of the smoke detectors to ensure sensitivity.
- Have working flashlights throughout the home (e.g., near the bed, in the kitchen, and in the basement). You can use the flashlight for evacuation or to signal for help.
- Know how to use the fire extinguisher before a fire occurs.
    - Every kitchen should have a fire extinguisher.
    - Always read the instructions so you will know how to use the extinguisher if necessary.
    - The International Association of Fire Chiefs (IAFC) recommends a multi-purpose or all-purpose extinguisher.
- Many new buildings are equipped with sprinkler systems; check for maintenance service.

3. Practice fire drills.
- If you do not practice, family members may not escape quickly enough.
- Designate a safe meeting place outside the home.
- Determine how you would safely transport the client out of the home, and discuss your plan with your supervisor. For example, one strategy might be using the bed linens for leverage and pulling the client to safety.
- If the client cannot walk, crawling down the stairs may be necessary.
- Practice the method with the client.
- Clients who have difficulty ambulating should have access to a telephone near the bed to call for help.

Contact your local fire department to see if programs are available to better accommodate homebound clients. Some departments use the "Find a Tot" sticker in the windows to help locate clients who may need more assistance.

Fire Safety in the Kitchen

Most fires occur in the kitchen. The following are tips to keep you safe in the kitchen.
- Turn off the range or stove when you leave the cooking area.
- Keep children away from the range and stove.
- Dress appropriately for cooking. Wear short or tight-fitting sleeves.
- Do not lean over the stove for items. Store items elsewhere. Cabinets above the range should not contain items that you need while cooking.

- Do not store flammable items (e.g., oven mitts, aerosol cans) near the heat.
- Keep the cooking area clean to prevent grease fires.
- Unplug appliances when not in use.
- Always have oven mitts and lids readily available in the event of a small pan fire (to smother the flames).
- If you are using burner covers on the stove, always remove all the covers to prevent accidental fires. It is easy to turn on the wrong burner and start a kitchen fire.
- Do not carry a pan on fire to the sink; it can ignite your clothing.
- If you have a fire in the oven, turn off the heat and keep the door closed (to suffocate the flames).
- If you have a fire in the microwave, turn off the power and unplug the unit.
- Always call the fire department if the fire does not go out.

Heater Fire Safety

The second leading cause of fires and fire deaths is faulty heating systems. Always follow the manufacturer's recommended maintenance program.

Portable and Space Heaters

- Place the heating unit at least 36 inches away from anything flammable (e.g., wallpaper, clothing, bedding, and people).
- Never leave the unit on if you are not in the room.
- Do not leave the unit on while sleeping.

Fireplaces

- Have the chimney inspected regularly. Creosote is a chemical substance that forms when wood burns. This can build up in the chimney and cause a fire.
- Use a sturdy screen in front of the fire.
- Never burn paper or pine branches; they can float out of the chimney and ignite your roof or adjacent homes.

Wood-Burning Stoves

- Treat wood-burning stoves the same as a space heater.
- Follow the manufacturer's recommended maintenance.

What to Do in a Fire

Knowing what to do in the event of a fire can save your life. Education is the best form of safety. Use the following techniques for fire safety.

1. At the first sign of fire, close the door to the room of the fire and exit the building.
2. Do not stop for anything, including gathering money, jewelry, pictures, or getting dressed.
3. Do not use the elevator.
4. If the room is smoky, cover your mouth with a towel or scarf (moistened if possible). This reduces the heat when breathing in the hot air.
5. Crawl or move as close to the floor as possible (where it is easier to breathe). Heat and smoke rise.
6. Feel the door for heat with the back of your hand before opening any doors.
   - If the door is hot to the touch, do not open it. Find an alternate exit.
   - If the door is cool, open it cautiously. Hold on to the door handle with one hand and, with the same-side back shoulder, slowly push the door open. Be prepared to shut the door quickly if you see smoke or flames.
7. When out of the building safely, call for help. Do not re-enter the building.
8. Stay with your client.
9. Keep yourself and your client as warm and comfortable as possible until help arrives.
10. Notify the agency as soon as possible.

Many apartment buildings and high-rises may have their own evacuation plan. Check with the building's superintendent or building manager.

AUDIENCE INTERACTION FOR TRANSPARENCY MASTER 2-2

Ask the audience to identify two ways of getting out of a building. Discuss scenarios of how to safely exit a building.

FIRE SAFETY QUESTIONS AND ANSWERS

Question: If I cannot get the client out of the house, what do I do?

Answer: If you cannot remove the client safely, exit the building and call for help. Alert others that the client is still in the building.

Question: If it is an apartment building, am I responsible for getting everyone out?

Answer: You are morally responsible for trying to alert others. Try yelling "fire" or pulling fire alarms.

Question: What if the exit is blocked by fire?
Answer:
- Remain calm.
- Look at your surroundings in every direction. Look for a fire escape or escape ladders.
- Do not jump out the window of a multi-story building.
- Call for help.

Question: What if there is no exit?
Answer:
- Seal off the fire by closing the door.
- Place a wet towel under the door to prevent smoke from entering the room.
- Stay close to the ground because the air is easier to breathe.
- Try to alert others that you are trapped by signaling at the window, for example, using a flashlight.

Question: If the fire is small, should I attempt to put it out?
Answer: Paying close attention to the environment can prevent common cooking fires. Fire extinguishers can put out small fires. Smothering the fire with a lid or pouring salt on the flames can easily put out grease fires.
- Never use water on a grease fire. The water may splatter the flames, which can ignite the surrounding area.
- Remember that fires can get out of control quickly and easily, so call for help.

● OXYGEN SAFETY

Oxygen is flammable and can easily be ignited. Special safety precautions must be taken when oxygen is in use.
- Do not smoke in the same room with the oxygen tank, even if the oxygen is not in use.
- Keep oxygen tanks away from heaters, stoves, electrical outlets, candles, and other items that can produce sparks.
- If possible, avoid wool or nylon. Use materials, such as cotton, that do not produce static electricity. Static electricity can produce sparks. Do not brush the client's hair when the oxygen is in use.
- The supervisor or the company distributing the oxygen should instruct the HCA and the client on oxygen safety.

- Contact your local fire department for more information.

General Lecture Material
No Transparency Master

SAFETY IN THE HOME

The home should be a safe environment, not only for the residents, but also for visitors. Make your home safe for everyone and keep your client's home safe.

AUDIENCE INTERACTION FOR GENERAL LECTURE MATERIAL

At a client's home, I was going to the bathroom to wash my hands when I felt a cord around my neck. I stepped back to find an extension cord reaching from the client's bedroom to the closet, five feet off the ground. The client needed a light in the closet, so she ran an extension cord from her bedroom. The client knew that it would be dangerous to have the cord on the ground, where someone could trip, so she had her son run it overhead. The client was not very tall and easily walked underneath it.

In this example, what are some of the hazards that can cause injuries?
- The electrical cord can cause neck injuries and make someone fall.
- Damage to an extension cord can cause sparks, fires, or electrocution.
- The light in the closet can catch on fire.

Burns
- Check the water temperature with your elbow or the inside of your wrist before bathing the client, to avoid scalding.
- Set water temperature on the water heater at 120°F.
- Use oven mitts when cooking.
- Keep handles of pots and pans turned away from the edge of the stove to prevent accidents.

Poisons
- Store cleaning supplies and poisons away from food.
- Keep poisons, cleaning supplies, and medications out of the reach of children.
- Read the labels on all items before use.
- Follow the directions on the label regarding "in case of accidental swallowing" or "in case of contact to eyes."
- Have poison control listed as one of the emergency telephone numbers. Check the telephone book for your local listing.

Common Household Hazards
- Area and scatter rugs can cause falls. Rugs must have rubber backing or be taped to the floor to prevent slipping.

- Loose banisters or no banisters in the stairway can cause clients to easily lose their balance when using the stairs.
- Poorly maintained stairs can cause clients to lose their footing and fall.
- Unsafe hallways, floors, and walls can cause clients to trip or fall. Falling can cause fractures and other serious injuries.
- Deteriorating ceilings can result in falling debris and cause head injuries.
- Poorly maintained stoves, appliances, electrical wiring, and heating can increase the risk of fire or electrocution.
- Wet floors can lead to the client's falling and possibly breaking a hip or other body part.
- Clutter in hallways or walk areas can prevent a timely escape in case of fire as well as be a risk factor for falls.

Lecture Material for Transparency Masters 2-3 and 2-4

FALLS

In the United States, one of every three adults, 65 years or older, falls each year (National Center for Injury Prevention and Control [NCIPC], 2000). In 2000, 10,273 people over the age of 65 died due to injuries from falls (WISQARS™, 2000).

- Falls are sometimes caused by hazards that can be easily fixed by:
  - securing scatter rugs and area rugs.
  - tightening loose banisters or installing banisters on staircases.
  - removing clutter from all walkways.
- Risk factors for falls include:
  - unsteady gait and balance.
  - neurologic and musculoskeletal limitations.
  - medication use.
  - dementia.
  - visual changes.

Fall Prevention

- Assist by moving items closer to the client.
- Avoid stairs. If there is no other option, use stairs cautiously.
- Create a regular exercise program to improve strength and coordination.
- Review medications, especially if the client is experiencing dizziness.
- Store medications in correctly labeled containers and keep out of the reach of children. All expired medications should be discarded.

- Have routine eye exams to detect:
  - glaucoma.
  - cataracts.
  - diabetes.
  - aging eyes.
- Wear properly fitting shoes.
- Encourage the proper use of assistive devices.
- Remove hazards by:
  - securing throw rugs.
  - installing banisters on stairways.
  - lighting all areas of the home.
  - removing clutter in passageways where falls or injuries can occur.
  - using a bathmat and installing a grab bar in the bathroom. Most accidents occur in the bathroom on wet, slippery floors.
  - avoiding unstable step stools. Make sure the step stool is secure. Test it to make sure it is sturdy enough to hold your weight before standing on it.
  - never standing on chairs or boxes. If your inner voice (common sense) tells you not to stand on an item, do not. Chairs are designed to withstand weight over the entire seat. When you stand on a chair, the weight is not evenly distributed and the chair can break or tip. Use step stools with handrails.

Other Risks for Falls

- Remember, standing in the shower can cause weakness, dizziness, or light-headedness.
- Falls can also be a result of nausea, vomiting, and diarrhea, which can cause changes in blood pressure, leading to dizziness or fainting.

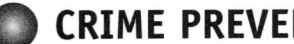 CRIME PREVENTION

Crime and violence are very much a part of our lives. For the HCA, the workplace is the community. This leads to an even greater risk for workplace violence. The HCA works alone and often works in high-crime areas. Most HCAs work in environments where they have little or no control.

Workplace Violence

Health care and social service settings have the highest incidence of workplace violence. The Occupational Safety and Health Administration (OSHA) and the National Institute of Occupational Health and Safety (NIOHS) define violence as "any physical assault, threatening behavior, or verbal abuse occurring in the workplace."

Perpetrators of Violence

Remember that everyone has the potential for violence. Violence can occur between:

- Employee and supervisor.
- Employee and employee.
- Employee and client or client's family.
- Employee and employee's family member (e.g., acts of domestic violence occurring at the workplace).
- Employee and stranger (e.g., robberies, shootings, muggings, drug seekers).

Misconceptions of workplace violence include the following:

- Many health care workers believe that acts of violence from clients are part of the job, especially with clients who cannot help their behavior because of confusion or medications.
- Many do not believe that resistance when bathing or changing clients or combativeness is considered violence.
- Health care workers believe that the clients cannot help themselves. Acting out and projecting their anger onto the health care worker is the clients' only coping mechanism.

Potential Issues With the Family or Client

- The client or client's family demands that the HCA perform duties that are not on the care plan.
- The client or client's family is not being kind to each other or the HCA.
- The client or client's family or friends make inappropriate comments or threats to the client or HCA.

Possible Triggers to Violence

- The disease or illness
- Client limitations
- Effects of certain medications
- Low self-esteem or personal problems (e.g., money, family members)
- Lack of support systems
- Mental illness

When accepting a case, ask the supervisor if the client has a history of "acting out."

- Have there been any previous reports of violence?
- Have there been any recent changes in the client's life (moves, medications, deterioration of illness, deaths)?

AUDIENCE INTERACTION FOR TRANSPARENCY MASTER 2-5

Dealing With Arguments

What should the HCA do if a client is arguing with him or her? (Insert your agency policy here.)

Answers:

- Never argue with the client.
- Make sure the client is safe.
- Remain calm (count to ten, leave the room, take deep breaths).
- Tell the client or client's family that you are offended, that you do not wish to be spoken to in that manner, and that you are going to leave if it continues.
    - If your performance is the issue, have the client call the agency or call the agency yourself.
    - If the client is unable to calm down, leave and report to the agency.
- Notify the supervisor of the first incident. It is easier to "nip it in the bud."
- At times, the hostile environment may be due to personality clashes. Changes in staff may be the best solution.

Ask the audience to name some acts of violence that an HCA may see in the home.

Answers:

Shouting	Kicking	Biting
Throwing items	Use of profanity	Pushing
Clients exposing themselves	Clients touching HCA inappropriately	Inappropriate comments

Ask the audience when these acts of violence should be reported.

Answer: Immediately

Discuss a common incident that can occur in the home.

Answer: A client exposes himself or herself to an HCA. The HCA gives up the case, stating another reason. The client exposes himself or herself to the replacement HCA. What was the responsibility of the previous HCA?

- Notify the supervisor.
- If you do not report the incident, the cycle will continue and the acts of violence may increase.

Lecture Material for Transparency Masters 2-6, 2-7, and 2-8

Potential Warning Signs of Violence

Observe all behaviors; violence can be prevented. Everyone has the potential for violence. Potential warning signs for violence include the following:

- Client talks about weapons or having weapons.
- Client makes threats.
- Client has no support systems.
- Client exhibits paranoid behaviors.

Transparency Master 2-7

- Client blames problems on others.
- Client experiences personal problems (e.g., financial, family).
- Client abuses drugs or alcohol.
- Client has a history of violence.
- Client was recently hospitalized for mental illness.
- Client reports suicidal or homicidal thoughts.

Transparency Master 2-8

- Client exhibits violent behaviors (e.g., yelling, screaming, and throwing items).
- Client undergoes changes in personality.

Discuss any fears you may have about the client or a client's family member with the supervisor, even if you cannot substantiate them. Gut feelings are important.

How to Prevent or Cope With Violence

- Be cautious.
- The HCA and agency staff must be proactive when dealing with violence. ("Better to be safe than sorry.")
- Set limits with the client and family members.
- Many employees overlook signs of violent behavior. Be aware of potential warning signs of violence and notify the supervisor.
- If the client or family member is showing signs of stress or violence, report it to the supervisor.
- If the HCA does not report the incident, no one will be able to help the client or HCA. Failure to report an incident can put other workers at risk.
- No one should have to be exposed to violence.
- Remember, risks of violence can come from:
  - clients or family members.
  - unsafe environments.
  - domestic problems.
  - coworkers.

*General Lecture Material
No Transparency Master*

SAFETY IN THE FIELD

Always be aware of your surroundings, especially of what is behind you. Pay attention to people around you.

- High-crime areas are not the only areas where crimes can occur. Always keep up your guard.
- Walk with an attitude.
- Remember that you are more important than any item. If a criminal approaches you and wants your purse or wallet, give it to him.
- Carry only the items you need.
  - Carry only enough money for that day. Do not carry large amounts of money if you do not plan on spending it.
  - Carry only the keys you need. Have your house and other keys on a separate key chain.
  - Your wallet should not have anything in it that cannot be replaced. Any keepsakes should be left at home. Carry only the necessary personal items.
  - Do not carry your social security card with you.

Learn How to Recognize, Avoid, and Defuse Potentially Violent Situations

General Measures

- Always walk in areas that are open and public; do not take shortcuts through alleys or behind buildings.
- Know where you are going. Call ahead to get directions.
- Walk with an attitude. If the criminal believes you are weak, you are going to be an easier target than someone who is walking proud.
- Get someone's attention if you feel threatened; yell "fire" or "money."
- Have your key ready when entering your home or car. The time it takes to find a key is enough time for a criminal to attack you.
- If you feel uncomfortable in an area, get out of there.
- Make others aware of where and when you are going, so they can keep an eye out for you.

Carrying Handbags

- Carry your belongings close to you. Do not swing your bag or dangle it from your shoulders. The criminal can run behind you and pull it off.
- Avoid wearing your bag sideways around your neck and shoulder. If a criminal tries to grab it, you will be pulled with it.
- The best way to carry a handbag is under your coat or jacket, and keep money in your pocket.
- If possible, do not carry a bag; keep all items in your pocket.

- Store your bag in the trunk of your car. Remember to place the bag in the trunk before arriving at your destination; otherwise, onlookers may break into your trunk and steal the bag.
- Always give the criminal what he wants. No money or jewelry is worth more than your life.
- Try carrying your bag upside down and under your arm. If the criminal tries to grab it, the bag will fall and all the items will fall out as well. The criminal is not going to stop and pick up the items.
- If you are approached by the criminal, run in the opposite direction. If the criminal grabs your bag, run in the opposite direction.

Car Safety

- Always lock your doors.
- Always wear your seat belt and have children restrained appropriately (in a car seat).
- Park your car in well-lighted areas. Try to avoid parking near concealed areas where criminals can hide (such as large bushes).
- If possible, have someone walk you to your car or watch you get into your car.
- Make sure you have enough fuel and your car is running properly.
- Before entering your car, look in the back seat and under your car. Criminals may hide under or in the car, wait for the door to open, then come out and steal the car or attack the victim in the car.
- When stopped, leave enough room between you and the car in front so that you can drive away if someone approaches.
- Do not place valuables or handbags in view because criminals may try to steal them from the car. Place them in the trunk of the car or under the seat.

Riding the Bus

- Be prepared and know the appropriate route.
- Wait at the designated bus stops, not in secluded areas.
- Stay alert and be aware of your surroundings.
- Do not get off in areas unfamiliar to you.
- If you feel uncomfortable on the bus, sit closer to the bus driver.

Dogs

According to the Centers for Disease Control and Prevention, an estimated 4.7 million people are bitten by dogs each year.

General Information

The following are facts provided by the American Veterinary Medical Association.

- All dogs are capable of biting.
- In the United States, 15 to 20 deaths per year are due to dog attacks.
- Never leave a baby or small child alone with a dog.
- Do not approach strange dogs.
- Ask permission from a dog's owner before petting the dog. Ask if the dog is friendly.
- Do not walk on a stranger's property.
- Do not pet the area on top of the head or the back of the neck. A dog might perceive this as a threat (it cannot see what you are doing). Instead, pet the underside of the dog's neck.
- Do not approach a dog if the dog is eating, sleeping, or caring for puppies.
- Always speak to the dog in soft tones.

Safe Behavior When Approached by a Dog
- Stay calm, do not scream, and remain still.
- Let the dog sniff you. Most dogs will sniff you and walk away. Do not run, because the dog will think it is a game and run after you.
- Avoid eye contact. Stand your ground.
- Do not bend down to pet the dog.
- Slowly back away from the dog or wait until the dog turns away.

Signs of Aggression
- The dog may growl or snarl. If the dog begins to growl and snarl (show teeth), stay calm.
- The dog will show its lips or teeth.
- The hair stands up on the dog's back.

Actions to Take When Bitten
- Do not pull away from the dog (the wound will tear).
- Thrust forward; the dog will need to get a better grip and will briefly release.
- Give something else to the dog to bite.
- Always protect your face and throat.
- If you are on the floor, crouch into a ball and cover your head and neck.

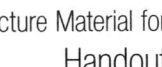

Lecture Material for Handout 2-3

 HOME-VISIT SAFETY

Always be sure of the address and directions to the case. Wear your uniform. Even in high-crime areas, the community usually looks after health care staff. Many times they watch out for the HCA because you are caring for their family.

- Always have your work identification card.
- Clients are told to look at the ID before letting the HCA inside.
- If you are in a high-crime area and the police enter the building to arrest members of the home, having the ID will verify to the police that you are there working as an HCA.
- Carry only what you need. Do not carry anything that appears to be a medical bag, so would-be thieves will not think you have any kind of medication, drugs, or needles.
- Do not enter a home if you do not have a description of the home or if there is no number on the client's home.
- Always use the elevators.
  - Stairways are sometimes secluded and criminals can hide out there.
  - Try to wait for an empty elevator if possible.
  - When entering an elevator, push a few of the floor buttons. In the event you feel uncomfortable, you can exit at the next floor. The persons on the elevator will not know on which floor you are exiting.
- If you feel threatened, never push the emergency stop button. You will become trapped with the person who is a threat.
- If the elevator is out of order, call the supervisor.
- Do not go down unlighted hallways or passageways.
- If your client is in a high-crime area, have the client or a family member look out the window for you, and have them call the agency if you are late.
- Keep to the assigned schedule; do not change it without notifying the supervisor. The assignments enable office staff to know where you are.
- If you feel uncomfortable entering a building because of a large group of people at the entrance to a client's home, do not go in. Call the agency.
- Any time you feel unsafe while at the client's residence:
  - try to do what is essential for the client and leave. If this is not possible, leave immediately.
  - report to your supervisor.
- If a client or client's family member makes threats, notify your supervisor at once.
- If the client is confused and makes a threat, even if you do not believe the client will act upon the threat, report it to your supervisor. The well-being of the HCA is important, and no threats should be treated lightly.
- Know the important telephone numbers, including the office or agency, client's home, police, and fire department.

General Lecture Material
No Transparency Master

FRAUD

Be on the lookout for other types of criminals. The ill and elderly are common targets of fraud. Keep your clients aware of fraudulent acts.

- Be aware of any offers that are too good to be true.
- Do not let anyone into the home unless without proper identification. If unsure, call the company and verify his or her employment. This includes:
    - meter readers.
    - public utilities (gas, electric, oil, phone, cable).
    - other HCAs, nurses, and social workers.
- When approached by a tradesperson, ask for references and proof of insurance. Never pay in full before the job is complete. Get more than one quote for a job.
- If you receive a bill in the mail and you are not familiar with the company, investigate before paying.
- Telemarketing fraud is especially common among elderly or homebound clients because clients:
    - may be lonely and enjoy talking to others.
    - may believe that the caller is just trying to make a living.
    - may not believe it is a crime, just a pushy salesperson.
    - have little money and want to believe that the deal is legitimate.

Signs that a solicitation could be telemarketing fraud include the following examples:

- Companies demand an immediate decision. Lawful businesses will always send more information about their company.
- Contests or sweepstakes promise elaborate gifts and then ask for money. True contests or sweepstakes do not ask for money because it is against the law.
- Investments are said to be risk-free. All investments have some risk and should be explained to the buyer carefully.
- Companies request cash only or payments wired directly to them.
- Companies ask for your social security number. Only if you are applying for credit should anyone ask you for your social security number. Be very careful to whom you give your social security number. A criminal can obtain credit cards by using your name and social security number, then steal your credit and identification. You may be responsible for some of the fraudulent bills or have to pay for a lawyer to represent you.
- Someone asks for your home address. Do not give it unless the caller is verified. Ask for a number where you can call him or her back.
- Be wary of charities requesting donations. Know the specific organization you are pledging. Many criminals pose as representatives

from organizations with similar names. (e.g., the Police Benevolent Society instead of the Police Benevolent Association).

- Collection agencies call to request payments for companies you have never heard of.

 ## AUDIENCE INTERACTION FOR GENERAL LECTURE MATERIAL

Thieves and criminals are very inventive. Ask the audience if they are aware of any other fraudulent acts. Discuss and describe:

- Investing in a fake investment.
- Asking for ID when workmen come to your home for repairs.
- Receiving a bill from a phony company.

For more information, contact the National Fraud Information Center at 1-800-876-7060.

Instructor's version with answers for Handout 2-2

 ## REAL-LIFE SCENARIO

A teenager arrived in the emergency department with complaints of light-headedness, headache, and disorientation. The patient stated that she had a headache and had taken four aspirins in two hours and was concerned that she may have taken too many pills. The bottle of pills was labeled aspirin. The medication inside was strong heart pills belonging to the patient's mother. The mother had placed the heart pills in the aspirin bottle for easy carrying. The teenager was admitted to the critical care unit.

Question 1. Where should the medication have been kept?

Answer: In the original bottle to prevent mistakes.

Question 2. If there was a problem with the original bottle, what other options could have been taken?

Answer: The mother could have put the medicine in a different bottle and labeled it with the correct name.

Question 3. What could have resulted from taking the incorrect medication?

Answer: Taking the incorrect medication can result in illness, disability, or death.

DEMONSTRATIONS

● PROPER WAY TO STAND

Demonstrate the following to the audience.
- For proper alignment, the body is straight but not tense.
- The feet face forward in the same direction as the knees.
- The legs are straight, but not tensed.
- The spine is long.
- The curves of the spinal column are within normal limits (the "S" shape is maintained).
- The head is upright.

● PROPER WAY TO TRANSFER A CLIENT FROM WHEELCHAIR TO CHAIR

1. Explain the procedure to the client.
2. Make sure the wheelchair is in the locked position.
3. Position the wheelchair at a 45-degree angle.
   a. Make sure the stronger side of the client faces the new location.
   b. The client can use the extremities of the stronger side to assist in the transfer.
   c. If it is unrealistic to transfer the client on the stronger side because of the floor plan of the home, transfer the client in the safest manner possible.
4. Keep both feet flat on the floor.
5. Spread your legs hip-width apart (about 10" to 12") for a broad base of support. If using the athletic stance, one foot should be in front of the other.
6. Face the client (no twisting).
7. Ask the client to slide to the edge of the chair and lean forward about 20 degrees.
8. Make sure the client's feet are flat on the floor.
9. Bend your knees.
10. Place your arms under the client's arms and lock hands together around the client.
11. On the count of three, have the client stand using the arms of the chair for leverage.
12. Hold the client and lift by straightening the knees. The largest and strongest muscles of the legs (quadriceps femoris) do the lifting.
13. Maintain the natural "S" curve of the back.
14. Instruct the client to take steps toward the chair. Use a rocking motion.
15. Move or pivot your feet, leading the client to the chair, but continue at the client's pace. (Do not twist the back.)

16. Ask the client to tell you when she feels the seat of the chair hit the back of her knees.

17. Bend and place the client into the chair, maintaining hold as she slides to the back.

18. Do not let go of the client until she is securely in the chair.

GROUP ACTIVITY

1. Ask the audience for volunteers to share what they have in their purse or wallet. (Have a sample bag available if you do not want a volunteer.) Empty out the items and determine whether they are safe to be in there. Determine whether a criminal can use an item against the victim, or if the victim will not be able to replace it.
   - Wallet with money can be replaced.
   - Driver's license can be replaced.
   - Good-luck charm given by grandmother who has passed away cannot be replaced.
   - Photo of your mother when she was a girl cannot be replaced.

2. Ask the audience to name some common hazards found in the home. Discuss responses.
   - Loose rugs
   - Loose railings
   - Dark hallways
   - Faulty heating systems
   - Frayed electrical wires

3. Review the checklist in Handout 2-4 to see if your home passes the safety test. The home-safety checklist can be used as a handout or overhead depending on the teaching strategy.

RESOURCES

American Veterinary Medical Association, *Tips to prevent being bitten.*
http://www.avma.org/

National Fire Protection Association
http://www.nfpa.org/

National Institute for Occupational Safety and Health
http://www.cdc.gov/niosh/homepage/

REFERENCES

Centers for Disease Control and Prevention. (2000, October). National Center for Injury Prevention and Control. *Falls and hip fractures among older adults.* Retrieved December 9, 2000, from http://www.cdc.gov/ncipc/factsheets/falls.htm

Fire safety and education. Retrieved November 27, 2000, from http://www.usfa.fema.gov/dhtml/public/facts.cfm

Gates, D. (1999). Violence against caregivers in nursing homes: Expected, tolerated and accepted. *Journal of Gerontological Nursing, 25*(4), 12–24.

Jacobs, J. (2000). Preventing workplace violence. *Surgical Services Management, 6*(5), 42–53.

Mills, D. (2000). Nurses fail to report workplace violence. *OHS Canada, 16*(7), 10.

National Consumers League National Fraud Information Center. (2000). *They can't hang up, help for elderly people targeted by fraud.* Retrieved December 3, 2000, from http://www.fraud.org/elderfraud/hangup.htm

National Fire Protection Association. (1998). *Fire loss in US & fire in the US, 1987–1996 Edition.* Author.

National Institute for Occupational Health and Safety. (1996). *Violence in the workplace: Risk factors and prevention strategies* (Current Intelligence Bulletin 56). Washington, DC: United States Department of Health and Human Services.

Occupational Safety and Health Administration. (1996). *Workplace violence awareness and prevention* (Fact Sheet No. OSHA 96-53). Washington, DC: United States Department of Labor.

WISQARS™. (2000). *Unintentional Fall Deaths and Rates per 100,000.* Hyattsville, MD: NCHS Vital Statistics System. Retrieved January, 2003, from http://webapp.cdc.gov/cgi-bin/broker.exe.

Name _____ Date _____

Program/Course _____ Instructor's Name _____

SAFETY
Pre/Post Test

1. Where do most home fires occur?
   a. kitchen
   b. living room
   c. basement
   d. fireplace

2. What type of accident in the home causes the most people over the age of 65 to be hospitalized?
   a. medication errors
   b. falls
   c. burns
   d. cuts

3. The following are part of home-safety guidelines. Which statement is *not* true?
   a. Emergency numbers should be posted near the telephone.
   b. Using electrical tape can repair frayed electrical cords.
   c. Throw rugs (area rugs) should be securely fastened to the floor.
   d. Store all medications out of reach of children.

4. Workplace violence can occur between:
   a. Employee and employee.
   b. Employee and family member.
   c. Employee and client or client's family.
   d. All of the above.

5. To live in society safely, we must learn how to recognize, avoid, or defuse potentially violent situations. Which of the following best describes that statement?
   a. Walk in areas that are open and public.
   b. Walk with an attitude.
   c. If you feel threatened, leave the area.
   d. All of the above

Handout **2-1**

Copyright © 2005 by Delmar Learning, a division of Thomson Learning, Inc.

Name _____ Date _____

Program/Course _____ Instructor's Name _____

REAL-LIFE SCENARIO

A teenager arrived in the emergency department with complaints of light-headedness, headache, and disorientation. The patient stated that she had a headache and had taken four aspirins in two hours and was concerned that she may have taken too many pills. The bottle of pills was labeled aspirin. The medication inside was strong heart pills belonging to the patient's mother. The mother had placed the heart pills in the aspirin bottle for easy carrying. The teenager was admitted to the critical care unit.

Question 1. Where should the medication have been kept?

Question 2. If there was a problem with the original bottle, what other options could have been taken?

Question 3. What could have resulted from taking the incorrect medication?

Handout **2-2**

HOME-VISIT SAFETY

1. Know where you are going.
   * Get directions.
   * Learn the area.
   * Know the bus route.
   * Always keep up your guard regardless of the area or location.
2. Always be aware of your surroundings.
3. Walk with an attitude. If the criminal believes you are weak, you are going to be an easier target than someone who is walking proud.
4. Wear your uniform and ID.
5. Carry only the items you need.
   * Work-related items (gloves)
   * Driver's license
   * Keys to your car
   * Only enough money for that day
6. Do not enter a home if there is no house number. Call to confirm building description.
7. Always use the elevators.
   * Stairways have many areas for a criminal to hide or jump out.
   * Push other floor buttons so you have the opportunity to leave the elevator if threatened.
   * Never push the emergency stop button if you feel threatened. You will be trapped with the person who is a threat.
8. Always walk in areas that are open and public.
   * Do not take shortcuts through alleys or behind buildings.
   * Stay in well-lighted areas.
9. Keep to the assigned schedule.
   * Make others aware of where and when you are going, so they can keep an eye out for you.
10. If you feel unsafe, leave.
    * Notify the supervisor.
    * If threatened, call the office or agency.
    * Get someone's attention if you feel threatened; yell "fire" or "money."
    * *No threats should be taken lightly.*
11. Report all incidents and concerns.
12. Know important numbers: office/agency, client's home, police, and fire department.

HOME-SAFETY CHECKLIST

- [ ] 1. Are lamps, extension cords, and telephone cords placed out of the flow of traffic?
- [ ] 2. Are emergency numbers posted on or near the telephone?
- [ ] 3. Are electrical cords in good condition and not frayed or cracked? Are they overloaded?
- [ ] 4. Are the small rugs and runners slip-resistant?
- [ ] 5. Is there access to a telephone near the sleeping area? Is the telephone easily accessible?
- [ ] 6. Do you have an escape plan in effect? Are there two ways to exit?
- [ ] 7. Is there at least one smoke detector on each floor? Are they tested regularly?
- [ ] 8. Is there any exposed wiring? Do the outlets and switches have cover plates?
- [ ] 9. Are the light bulbs the appropriate size and shape for the lamps or fixtures?
- [ ] 10. Are small stoves, space heaters, and other heating sources away from flammable material?
- [ ] 11. Are towels, curtains, and other flammable materials located away from the range?
- [ ] 12. Are hallways, stairs, passageways between rooms, and other heavy-traffic areas well lighted? Are exits and passageways kept clear?
- [ ] 13. Are showers and bathtubs equipped with non-skid surfaces?
- [ ] 14. Do bathtubs and showers have at least one grab bar?
- [ ] 15. Are all medicines stored in proper containers and out of reach of children?
- [ ] 16. Are there banisters in the stairway? Are they secure?

SAFETY IN THE WORKPLACE

E.D.I.T.H.
Exit Drills In The Home

1. Create an escape plan.

2. Review the plan.

3. Practice fire drills.

Fall Prevention Checklist

✓ Use assistance when needed

✓ Use stairs cautiously

✓ Create a regular exercise program

✓ Review medications

(continues)

Fall Prevention Checklist
(continued)

✓ Have routine eye exams

✓ Wear proper shoes

✓ Use a cane/walker

✓ Remove hazards

Workplace violence is: "any physical assault, threatening behavior, or verbal abuse occurring in the workplace."

(From OSHA and the National Institute of Occupational Health and Safety)

Potential Warning Signs of Violence

- Talks about weapons/has weapons
- Makes threats
- Has no support systems
- Exhibits paranoid behaviors

(continues)

Potential Warning Signs of Violence
(continued)

- Blames problems on others
- Experiences personal problems
- Abuses drugs or alcohol
- Has a history of violence

(continues)

Potential Warning Signs of Violence
(continued)

- Was recently hospitalized for mental illness
- Reports suicidal or homicidal thoughts
- Exhibits violent behavoirs
- Undergoes changes in personality

Module 3
Abuse

GOAL

To identify, report, and help prevent abuse

OBJECTIVES

After completion of the presentation, students will be able to:
- List the types of child maltreatment.
- Discuss ways to control anger and frustration.
- Describe how to report child maltreatment.
- List the three categories of elder abuse.
- Describe signs of self-neglect.
- Describe how to report elder abuse.
- List four preventive measures to reduce abuse.
- Explain what is meant by domestic violence.

Lecture Material for Transparency Master 3-1

Each section of this module can be presented individually.

CHILD ABUSE

Abuse is more common than we are aware of and occurs in all walks of life.

⬤ GENERAL INFORMATION/OVERVIEW

- In 1999, the United States Department of Health and Human Services estimated that 2.9 million cases of child maltreatment were investigated.
  - 58.4% were victims of neglect.
  - 21.3% were physically abused.
  - 11.3% were sexually abused.
  - 35% were either abandoned or had threats of harm.
- The actual incidence of child abuse is likely to be higher than reported.
- Two-thirds of abused children are school aged, eight years old or older.
- 10% of emergency room visits account for injuries due to abuse of children under the age of 7.
- Children with disabilities are abused more frequently.
- Child abuse causes an estimated 2,000 deaths each year, or 5 children every day. The death rate actually may be higher because many of the deaths due to abuse or neglect are listed as accidents or homicides.
- A common precipitating event to abuse is a crying baby. Death occurs most often in children under the age of three.
- 57% of children murdered before age 12 are killed by a parent.

⬤ HISTORY

- Child abuse emerged as a topic of major medical concern in the early 1960s.
- Health professionals can detect signs of chronic and traumatic abuse in young children by documenting previous fractures, burns, and bruises in the form of healed injuries that are no longer visible.
- With this knowledge, the federal government has developed a national child-abuse reporting system. Mandatory reporting is the first component of the child protection policy.
- In 1976, the Child Abuse Prevention and Treatment Act (CAPTA) was signed. CAPTA defines child abuse and neglect with the following criteria:
  - The victim must be less than 18 years of age.
  - Abuse is any recent act or failure to act on the part of a parent or caretaker that results in death, serious physical or emotional harm, sexual abuse, or exploitation.

- Abuse is an act or failure to act that presents imminent risk of serious harm.
- Each state provides its own definition, reporting statutes, and interventions. Contact your state Child Protective Services for information regarding state definition and legislation.

- Some states have a broader definition of child abuse, which gives the Child Protective Services and the state more jurisdiction.

TYPES OF MALTREATMENT

Lecture Material for Transparency Master 3-2

Maltreatment or abuse takes on many forms. Incidents range from mild bruising to life-threatening injuries.

(Insert your state's definition of maltreatment here.)

Physical Abuse of Children

General Information

- Physical injury includes beating, burning, biting, kicking, shaking, and shoving.
- The abuser may not intend to harm the child, but the abuse results from excessive discipline or physical punishment.
- The caregiver often has no explanation, is inconsistent, or unconvincing when explaining the injury.
- The most common injuries due to physical abuse are head injuries and damage from blunt trauma.

Signs of Physical Abuse

Trauma Marks

- Markings may include bruises, welts, or lacerations on the back or abdomen, which can be concealed by clothing.
- Bruises in various stages of healing indicate repeated injuries.

Burns

- Burns may cause imprint marks indicated by the shape of the item used (e.g., irons, cigarettes).
- Immersion burns are caused by placing a body part into burning liquid.
  - Burns look like a sock over the feet and legs.
  - Burns look like a glove over the hands and arms.
  - Burns cover a round area over the buttocks and genitalia.

Fractures and Head Injuries

- Fractures in young children often include spiral fractures of the arms or legs, facial fractures, and rib fractures.
- Abuse may involve head injuries in children under two years of age that cannot be explained by trauma (such as motor vehicle accidents).
- Physicians should order a skeletal survey to look for old fractures if abuse is suspected.

Human Bites

- A human bite can occur on any area of the body.
- Human bites crush the tissues and cause tissue bruising, whereas animal bites tear the tissue.

Lecture Material for Transparency Master 3-3

Emotional Abuse in Children

General Information

Emotional abuse includes psychological, verbal, and mental abuse. It is difficult to prove because there is no physical evidence of harm to the child. Emotional abuse consistently occurs with other types of child maltreatment.

- Emotional abuse consists of acts by parents or caregivers including unreasonable demands, verbal attacks, and constant belittling of the child.
- Abuse includes extreme punishment such as confinement; belittling; constant teasing; rejection; and lack of love, support, or guidance.

Signs of Emotional Abuse

The child may:

- Be extremely demanding or obedient.
- Be very aggressive or very passive.
- Portray adult behaviors (e.g., parenting other children) or infantile behaviors.
- Be overly friendly to strangers.
- Show a delay in physical or emotional development (e.g., difficulty learning to talk).
- Have difficulty with close relationships.
- Have low self-esteem.
- Have problems in school.

Lecture Material for Transparency Master 3-4

Sexual Abuse in Children

General Information

Sexual abuse includes fondling, intercourse, incest, rape, sodomy, exhibitionism, and commercial exploitation through prostitution or the production of pornographic materials (National Clearinghouse on Child Abuse and Neglect Information, July 2000). The age that constitutes child abuse is specific for each state.

- Most sexual abuse is from a family member or trusted family friend.
- More girls are sexually abused (16%–34%) than boys (10%–20%).
- Victims remain loyal to their abusers even as adults.

Signs of Sexual Abuse

The child may:

- Display changes in behavior, such as sleeping.
- Become very secretive.
- Experience pain when walking or sitting.
- Develop a poor appearance.
- Display inappropriate sexual behavior or knowledge of sex.
- Be frightened by physical contact.
- Refuse to change for gym class or participate in physical activities.
- Run away.
- Become pregnant or contract a sexually transmitted disease (especially before the age of 14).

Lecture Material for Transparency Master 3-5

Child Neglect

Child neglect is the failure of the caregiver to provide for the child's basic needs. Neglect is most commonly seen in children under eight years of age.

Types of Neglect

Physical Neglect

- Refusal of or delay in seeking health care
- Abandonment
- Banishment from the home
- Custody issues
- Inattention to hazards in the home

Supervision Neglect

- Inadequate supervision
- No supervision
- Leaving a very small child in the care of a slightly older child

Emotional Neglect

- Inadequate affection
- Exposure to domestic violence
- Permitting substance abuse
- Permitting unfavorable behavior (chronic delinquency)
- Delay in or refusal of psychological treatment

Educational Neglect

- Truancy
- Failure to enroll in school
- Failure to provide for special needs

Inadequate Supervision

Inadequate supervision is the most common form of neglect-related deaths resulting from:

- Hazardous material exposure.
- Dangerous situations.
- Smoke inhalation.
- Drowning.
- Medical neglect.

Signs of Neglect

The child may:

- Have poor hygiene and be malnourished.
- Be inappropriately dressed for the weather.
- Lack adequate health care; for example:
  - frequently miss doctors' appointments.
  - lack or lose eyeglasses or hearing aids.
  - have no dental care.
  - be behind on immunizations.
  - frequently be absent from school.
  - perform poorly in school.
  - have sleep disturbances.
  - be depressed or anxious.
  - display aggressive behavior.
  - beg classmates for food or money or steal.
  - avoid going home.
  - have poor interpersonal relationships and prefer being alone.
  - use alcohol or drugs.

General Lecture Material No Transparency Master

CAUSES OF CHILD ABUSE AND NEGLECT

Characteristics of Abusers

The abuser may:
- Have limited coping skills and react to stress with violence.
- Be provoked by certain household members, resulting in uncontrolled anger.
- Have financial trouble.
- Experience changes in home life, such as divorce, relocation, or cohabitation with different people.
- Consider violence a normal behavior.

Anyone can be an abuser.
- Abuse can affect any family regardless of socioeconomic status, race, or culture.
- Abusers may have poor parenting skills and show disregard for the child's needs.
- The parents may be young and have poor coping skills. Abuse may occur after the birth of additional children.
- A study by Prevent Child Abuse of America stated that 50% of Americans with children reported that they found themselves in situations in which they feared they might abuse or neglect their child on more than one occasion. The study also noted that 15% feared that they might abuse or neglect their child very often.
- Many abusers have been victims of abuse themselves.
- Domestic violence increases the likelihood of child abuse.
- Drug and alcohol abuse increase the risk of child abuse.

Statistics on Abusers

The U.S. Department of Health and Human Services (*Child Maltreatment*, 1999) reported the following:
- 61.8% of the abusers are women.
- 87.3% of the abuse is by at least one parent.
- 3.9% are relatives.
- 1.5% are caregivers (e.g., health care workers, baby sitters, child care workers).
- 7.2% are other or unknown relationships.
- 80% of the abusers are under the age of 40.

There is a higher incidence of abuse in lower-income families because of the increased stresses from:
- Unemployment.
- Depression.

- Isolation.
- Substance abuse.
- Domestic violence.

Recognizing an Abuser

- The parent may show little concern or interest in the child's school performance or sports activities. Conversely, the parent may demand perfection from the child with regard to schooling, extracurricular activities, and household chores.
- The abuser blames the child for his or her problems and expresses dissatisfaction or disappointment in the child to others.
- The abuser looks to the child for support, attention, and emotional needs or may be indifferent about the child.

EFFECTS OF CHILD ABUSE AND NEGLECT

The effects of abuse vary among victims of child maltreatment. Abused children often bring the trauma into adolescence, adulthood, and parenthood. On the other hand, some abused children show few consequences in adulthood.

Several factors may influence the effects of the abuse:
- Intensity of the abuse
- Type of abuse
- Duration of the abuse
- The child's age at the time of the abuse
- The child's support systems

Some effects of the abuse are seen in the child's personality and behavioral development. Abused children are less likely to trust others and may have difficulty with interpersonal relationships, such as the parent/child relationship, relationships with peers, and intimate relationships, and may be prone to abusive relationships. Victims of abuse are more likely to be arrested and commit violent crimes.

Victims of sexual abuse have a higher risk for:
- Depression.
- Anxiety.
- Eating disorders.
- Addictions.
- Problems with sexual relations.

The following are possible behaviors of abused children:
- Feeling helpless, hopeless, and ashamed
- Depression
- Substance abuse

- Eating disorders
- Suicidal behavior
- Psychiatric disorders

REPORTING CHILD ABUSE AND NEGLECT

Each state designates who is mandated to report incidents of child abuse. Child victims do not disclose the abuse for the following reasons:

- Fear of the abuser
- Fear of negative reactions from family members
- Fear that no one will believe them
- Belief that they deserved the abuse
- They do not know the abuse is wrong.

(Insert your agency's policy for reporting abuse here.)

STEPS TO PREVENT CHILD MALTREATMENT

The harmful effects of abuse can be decreased with early intervention.

Tips for Parents

- Nurture your child with compliments for work well done and show interest in his/her hobbies.
- Offer to help a friend or neighbor care for the children so the parent(s) can rest. Being a parent is not easy.
- If you feel overwhelmed and out of control, make time for yourself and do not take it out on the children. Ask someone to watch the children so you can take a break.
- Ask the doctor what to do if your baby will not stop crying.
- If you find yourself getting frustrated and angry with your baby, call for help. Place the child in a safe place in the home (the crib) and shut the door. Never shake a baby because it can cause severe injury or death.
- Encourage community leaders, clergy, library, and schools to develop services to meet the needs of children and families.
- Report suspected abuse or neglect. Violence will increase in frequency and severity unless someone intervenes.

(Adapted from Prevent Child Abuse America. *Ten Ways to Help Prevent Child Abuse,* http://www.preventchildabuse.org.)

AUDIENCE INTERACTION FOR GENERAL LECTURE MATERIAL

Ask the audience to describe ways to control anger and frustration. Review each answer.

Tips to Control Anger and Frustration

Learning to control anger and frustration can help prevent child abuse. (Adapted from Prevent Child Abuse America. *Twelve Alternatives to Lashing Out at Your Child*, http://www.preventchildabuse.org.)

Use Relaxation Techniques

- Take deep breaths. Remember that you are the adult.
- Count to ten.
- Use imagery.

Take a Time-Out

- Close your eyes and imagine you are hearing what your child is about to hear.
- Put your child in time-out and remember the time-out rule: one time-out minute for each year of age.
- Put yourself in time-out and think about why you are angry. Is it your child, or is the child a convenient target for your anger?

Seek Respite

- Phone a friend.
- If someone can watch the children, go outside and take a walk.
- If someone cannot watch the children, place children in a safe place (such as the crib) and shut the door.
- Take a hot bath or splash cold water on your face.
- Hug a pillow.
- Turn on some music, and maybe even sing along.
- Pick up a pencil and write down as many helpful words as you can think of and save the list.
- Call for more information: 1-800-CHILDREN.

DOMESTIC VIOLENCE

Domestic violence is also known as spouse or partner abuse. Domestic violence is not just about losing your temper; it is about controlling someone. It is the most commonly unreported crime in the United States.

● GENERAL INFORMATION/OVERVIEW

Information is obtained from the U.S. Department of Justice, Office of Justice Programs web site (http://www.ojp.usdoj.gov/vawo/welcome.htm) and The National Council on Child Abuse and Family Violence (http://www.nccafv.org).

- The U.S. Department of Justice estimates that 95% of reported assaults on spouses or ex-spouses are committed by men against women.
- Men are less likely to report abuse, so it is difficult to determine the extent of male victims. Abuse also can happen in same-sex relationships.
- Each year, an estimated 3 to 4 million women in the United States are abused by their male partners.
- According to the American Medical Association, domestic violence is the leading cause of injury and death to women in the United States.
- An estimated 3.3 million children annually are exposed to violence by family members against their mothers or female caregivers.
- Enforcement of crimes against women has been slow because of society's tolerant view of domestic violence.
- As with other types of abuse, victims feel ashamed and helpless and often do not report the violence.

Recent Legislation

The Violence Against Women Act (Title IV of the Violent Crime Control and Law Enforcement Act of 1994; P.L. 103-322) provides for grants to assist states to develop and strengthen effective law enforcement and prosecution strategies to combat violent crimes against women. It also develops and strengthens victim services involving violent crimes against women.

The Violence Against Women Act of 2000 improves legal tools and programs addressing domestic violence, sexual assault, and stalking.

TYPES OF DOMESTIC VIOLENCE

Physical Abuse

- Physical abuse is the most commonly reported form of domestic violence.
- Physical injuries result from slapping, punching, choking, biting, hair pulling, or shoving. Shoving is a warning sign of someone trying to control another person.

Sexual Abuse

The victims are hurt, degraded, dominated, or humiliated for the abuser to gain power over them. Acts of aggression and threats accompany the abuse. Abuse may consist of:

- Marital rape.
- Forced or coerced sexual acts.
- Unwanted fondling or intercourse.

Psychological Abuse/Emotional Abuse

Psychological and emotional abuse controls the victim's behavior and it damages self-esteem. It includes verbal abuse, interrogation, intimidation, and isolation.

Verbal Abuse

Verbal abuse includes verbal attacks, insults, or degrading remarks. This behavior is always present with other forms of abuse.

Threats of Abuse/Intimidation

The abuser threatens the victim in various ways. Most of the intimidating threats occur behind closed doors. The victim's fear is real even if others feel there is no threat. Examples of threats or acts of intimidation include:

- Threatening to hit, harm, or use a weapon on another person.
- Threatening to tell secrets or confidential information.
- Intimidating the victim with looks, actions, gestures, yelling, or smashing objects.
- Threatening to kill the victim's family or children. ("I will kill your sister if I find out you were with her.")
- Threatening to take away the children. ("If you go, you cannot take the children.")
- Threatening to commit suicide. ("I cannot live without you.")

Isolation

The abuser keeps his partner from people who are important to her, restricts her social events, or forbids her from leaving the home. Controlling all of the finances and preventing the partner from getting a job worsen the isolation.

CHARACTERISTICS OF A BATTERED WOMAN

- Battered women come from all walks of life, including every social, economic, religious, and racial group.
- Battered women often feel degraded and worthless and may feel that they deserve the mistreatment. Lack of positive self-esteem may keep her from telling anyone about the abuse or make her believe she is a failure as a wife and/or mother.
- The victim feels a duty to keep the family together, no matter what the cost. She may submit to the abuse for the sake of the children, and often leaves the relationship only when the violence becomes directed at the children.
- The victim keeps the abuse a secret and believes that society ignores domestic violence. She feels she will be blamed for provoking or accepting the violence.

- The victim is dependent on the spouse financially and often faces severe economic hardship if she leaves. She may have few job skills and be unable to support herself and the children.
- The victim feels isolated from family and friends. This gives the abuser more power and control.

CHARACTERISTICS OF THE ABUSER

No typical profile for men who batter has been identified. The abuser may exhibit the following behaviors:

- Denies the existence of violence
- Shows jealousy and extreme possessiveness of the partner
- Refuses to accept responsibility for the abuse, blaming the violence on stress, alcohol, drugs, or the victim
- Has a history of family violence
- Has a negative attitude toward women

FACTORS CONTRIBUTING TO ABUSIVE BEHAVIOR

- Men who batter choose to do so and, until recently, there has been no consequence for this behavior.
- Battering is a learned behavior, not a mental disorder. Abusers usually have a history of family violence. Witnessing domestic violence as a child is the most common risk factor for becoming an abuser in adulthood.
- Abusers learned to use physical force as a way to maintain power and control. Battering is the ultimate expression of the belief in male dominance over females.
- Physical violence is used as a coping mechanism. Abuse is the only way they can handle anger, frustration, or guilt because of their low self-control.
- Abusers lack the communication skills to handle emotions in nonviolent ways and usually displace their anger onto the partner.
- Abusers may seek forgiveness from the victim, promising it will never happen again. Such promises are rarely kept.
- Abusers have a negative attitude toward women/men.
- The abuse may stem from religious or cultural beliefs.
  - Mistreatment of family members, especially women, is common in some cultures. Those who participate in these behaviors do not consider them abuse.
  - In some cultures, women's basic rights are not honored. Older women in these cultures may not realize they are being abused. They probably could not go outside the family for help and may not even know that help is available.
- Violent behavior is seen in the entertainment industry and the media.
- The lack of public awareness that domestic violence is a crime contributes to the behavior.

SIGNS OF DOMESTIC ABUSE

- Injuries to and chronic pain in the face, neck, throat, chest, abdomen, or genitals.
- Injuries in various stages of healing
- Delays in treatment for injuries
- Injuries during pregnancy
- Inconsistent explanations for the causes of injury
- A partner who is overly aggressive

REASONS BATTERED WOMEN STAY

For many victims, leaving is not an option. The victims do not want to end the relationship, just the violence. Many victims are dependent on the perpetrator. Statistics show that the average battered woman leaves the relationship seven times before she leaves for good.

Leaving an abusive relationship is a process and one that is often long and drawn-out. This can be very frustrating for relatives and friends. The person who is in the abusive relationship is the only person who can decide when the time is right to leave. Respect the abused person's right to make his or her own decisions.

Fear

- The most dangerous time during an abusive relationship is when the victim tries to leave.
- Statistics estimate that 1,400 women in the United States die each year as a result of domestic violence.
- A woman may stay in the relationship, isolated from others, to protect her family from the abuser.
- The abuser may threaten anyone who is trying to help the victim leave the relationship.

Low Self-Esteem

- Beatings and intimidation cause women to no longer believe in themselves.
- Women believe that no one can help and they remain isolated from others.
- Women may believe that they deserve the violence.

Cycle of Violence
- The abuser states that it will not happen again.
- The abuser is very apologetic and loving after the violence.
- The abuser makes promises to the victim.
- The abuse may not happen frequently at first, but typically, the abuse worsens and the violence becomes more frequent.

Limited Resources
- The abuser is the main source of love and affection.
- The victim feels isolated from friends and family.
- The victim is financially dependent on the abuser and feels there is nowhere to go.

History of Family Violence
- The victim was raised in an abusive family.
- The victim may not be aware that abuse is an unacceptable behavior.

PREVENTING DOMESTIC VIOLENCE
Treat Domestic Violence as a Crime
- States need more effective laws governing domestic violence crimes, including simpler procedures for filing restraining orders.
- Domestic violence must be taken seriously, and the abusers must be arrested and convicted for their crimes.

Educate the Community
- Society needs to be educated on the effects violence has on women and children.
- Changing attitudes toward victims of domestic violence and their families is the first step.

Provide Community Services
- Shelters and counseling services must be made readily available to victims and their families.
- Attorneys and legal-aid programs need to increase services for battered women, including restraining orders, divorce, and custody issues.

If You Suspect Abuse, Notify Your Supervisor
- If the client confirms abuse, ask if she wants help and notify your supervisor.
- Do *not* make a promise not to reveal the abuse. The home may not be safe for you, and any form of violence must be reported to your supervisor.

Talk to the Victim

Let the victim know:
- There is no excuse for domestic violence.
- No one deserves abuse.
- It is not your fault.
- Help is available (e.g., support groups, shelters, and legal advice).

The National Domestic Violence Hotline provides information on how to find help in your community: 800-799-SAFE (7233), or 800-787-3224 (TDD) 24 hours a day.

Lecture Material for Transparency Master 3-8

ELDER ABUSE

More elderly people are living longer and are dependent on others for their care. Even if they are not in a high-risk group, the elderly can find themselves in abusive situations.

GENERAL INFORMATION/OVERVIEW

- For every case of elder abuse and neglect that is reported, experts believe there may be five cases that have not been reported.
- Elders who are ill, frail, disabled, mentally impaired, or depressed are at greater risk for abuse.
- Men and women over the age of 80 are two to three times more likely to be abused or neglected than the remaining elderly population.
- Older adults who have been abused tend to die sooner than those who are not abused, even in the absence of disease.

Elder abuse is more difficult to detect than child abuse because:
- Children over the age of 5 years go to school and have contact with other adults. The elderly do not.
- Approximately one-quarter of older adults live alone. Children do not live alone.
- Interaction is primarily with family members and very few outsiders. Children have outside interaction.
- Social isolation may increase the risk of maltreatment. Children live with their families and are not socially isolated.

HISTORY

Federal definitions of elder abuse, neglect, and exploitation appeared for the first time in the 1987 Amendments to the Older Americans Act (42 U.S.C. 3001 et seq., as amended). This amendment provides guidelines for identifying problems of elder abuse; it does not have any enforcement purposes.

- State laws define elder abuse, and state definitions vary in what constitutes abuse, neglect, or exploitation of the elderly.
- There are no federal laws for elder abuse equivalent to the federal laws on child abuse and no shelters for victims, as with domestic violence.

CATEGORIES OF ELDER ABUSE

Domestic Elder Abuse

- Domestic elder abuse includes any form of maltreatment of an older person by someone who has a special relationship with the elder (e.g., spouse, child, friend, or caregiver), living in the older person's own home or in the home of a caregiver.
- Domestic elder abuse includes physical, emotional, or sexual abuse; neglect; and abandonment. There is no single documented pattern of elder abuse in the home.

Institutional Elder Abuse

Institutional elder abuse refers to any of the previously mentioned forms of elder abuse that occurs in residential facilities, nursing homes, foster homes, group homes, or board and care. The abuse can include physical, emotional, or sexual abuse; neglect; and abandonment. The abusers can be persons who have a legal or contractual obligation to provide the elderly with care and protection (e.g., paid caregivers, staff, and professionals).

Self-Neglect or Self-Abuse

Self-abuse includes any behavior or action that threatens an older person's health or safety because of his or her own physical or psychological limitations.

TYPES OF ELDER ABUSE

Physical Abuse

The use of physical force may result in bodily injury, pain, or physical impairment. Examples of physical abuse are hitting, shoving, shaking, slapping, kicking, pinching, burning, inappropriate use of restraints (physical or chemical restraints/sedation), and force-feeding.

Signs of physical abuse include:

- Unkempt overall appearance of the client, such as poor hygiene or inappropriate dress for the season.
- Sudden changes in client's behavior that are not due to illness or medication.

- Bruises, especially where covered by clothing.
- Black eyes, broken eyeglasses or frames.
- Fractures.
- Cuts, lacerations, and welts.
- Untreated injuries in various stages of healing.
- Sprains and dislocations.
- Internal injuries and bleeding.
- Signs of being restrained (such as rope burns).

Emotional Abuse

Lecture Material for Transparency Master 3-10

Emotional abuse is mental or emotional distress caused by verbal or non-verbal acts, such as humiliation, intimidation, or harassment. The abuse isolates the elderly person from his family, friends, or regular activities.

Signs of emotional abuse include:
- Being emotionally upset or agitated.
- Being withdrawn and noncommunicative or unresponsive.
- Having difficulty sleeping.
- Displaying unusual behavior, such as sucking, biting, or rocking.
- Showing improvement of behavior when not in the care of the abuser.

Sexual Abuse

Lecture Material for Transparency Master 3-11

Sexual abuse is nonconsensual sexual contact of any kind or sexual contact with any person incapable of giving consent. This includes unwanted touching, all types of sexual assault and/or battery, coerced nudity, and sexually explicit photography.

Signs of sexual abuse include:
- Injuries around the breasts or genital area.
- Venereal disease without explanation.
- Vaginal or anal bleeding without explanation.
- Torn, stained, or bloody undergarments.
- Pain when walking or sitting.

Financial Abuse

Lecture Material for Transparency Master 3-12

Financial abuse is stealing or misusing money or property without the older adult's knowledge and for someone else's benefit. This may include:
- Cashing the person's checks without permission.
- Forging a signature.

- Misusing money or possessions.
- Coercing or deceiving an older person into signing a document (such as contracts or a will).
- Misusing guardianship or power of attorney.

Signs of financial abuse include:
- Changes in the elder person's bank account.
- Unexplained transfers of assets to a family member or someone outside the family.
- Unexplained withdrawal of large sums of money.
- Additional names on bank accounts.
- Unauthorized withdrawal of funds using the client's ATM card.
- Forged signatures for financial transactions or for the titles of possessions.
- Changes in the client's will.
- Bills unpaid despite ample financial resources.
- Payment for services that are not necessary (e.g., lawn service for a client living in an apartment).
- Valuables disappearing from the client's home.
- Uninvolved relatives claiming rights to the client's possessions.

Lecture Material for Transparency Master 3-13

Neglect

Neglect is the most common form of elder maltreatment. It is defined as the refusal or failure of a caregiver to provide basic needs for the elder, including food, clothing, shelter, and medical care. Neglect may also include:

- Failure to provide services necessary to avoid physical harm and mental anguish and ensure home safety.
- Failure of the person with fiduciary responsibilities to provide care for the older client. For example, the person with power of attorney refuses to pay for the necessary home care services.
- Failure of a paid in-home service provider to arrange necessary care. An example is when a home care aide (HCA) does not go to the scheduled case.

Signs of neglect include:
- Dehydration.
- Malnutrition.
- Inappropriate dress for weather conditions.
- Caregiver's refusal of visitors.
- Untreated pressure sores.
- Poor personal hygiene.
- Untreated health problems.

- Hazardous or unsafe living conditions or arrangements.
- Improper electrical wiring; no heat or running water.
- An unsanitary living condition, such as dirt, fleas, or soiled bedding.

Self-Neglect

Self-neglect includes any behavior or action that threatens an older person's health or safety because of his or her own physical or psychological limitations. It remains a serious problem because many elderly people are isolated.

- The client may be confused or physically debilitated.
- The client may refuse or fail to provide herself with adequate food, water, clothing, shelter, personal hygiene, medication, and safety precautions.
- Most cases of self-neglect involve women.
- 45% of self-neglect cases involve people over the age of 80 years.

The definition of self-neglect excludes a client who is mentally competent and understands the consequences of his or her decisions. No one can force competent adults to change the way they live, even if the acts can threaten their health or safety. The elderly have the right to determine their affairs to the full extent of their ability as long as they are deemed competent.

Signs of self-neglect include:
- The inability to manage personal finances by failure to pay bills, stashing money, or giving money away.
- The inability to maintain activities of daily living, including personal care, food shopping, meal preparation, housekeeping, and appropriate dress.
- The inability to maintain safety by wandering, refusing medical attention, leaving the stove on, and/or lack of security.
- An unsafe living environment, without utilities or working toilets or with faulty wiring.
- Homelessness.
- A declining health status with dehydration, malnutrition, and untreated illnesses.
- Changes in mental status with confusion, inappropriate responses, disorientation, and memory loss.
- Lack of medical interventions, such as eyeglasses; hearing aids; dentures; decayed, missing, and filled teeth; and regular doctor's appointments.

Abandonment

Abandonment is a form of neglect in which the caregiver leaves the elderly person with no intention of resuming the caregiver role.

- The elderly person can be left at a health care facility (e.g., hospital, nursing home, adult day care center).
- The caregiver refuses to pick up the client at the time of discharge and cannot be reached or contacted.
- The caregiver can "dump" the client at the emergency department of the hospital and not return.
- The caregiver may leave the elderly person at a public location (e.g., shopping center, library, parking lot, bus station).
- The caregiver no longer wants to accept responsibility for the client.
- The elderly person may be confused and unable to identify the caregiver or his residence.

CHARACTERISTICS OF ELDER ABUSERS

Adult children are most frequently the abusers of the elderly as compared with other family members. The abuser can also be an informal or formal caregiver.

There are several indicators of abuse from the caregiver. The caregiver or abuser may:

- Prevent the older adult from speaking.
- Be apathetic or angry toward the elderly person.
- Fail to assist the older adult with personal needs.
- Blame the client for accidents, such as accusations of deliberately spilling food or soiling the bed.
- Display aggressive behaviors (e.g., threats, insults, and harassment) toward the elderly person.
- Be overly affectionate around company or outsiders.
- Display inappropriate sexual behavior with the older adult.
- Restrict activities or isolate the client from family. Sometimes abusers will threaten to keep people away from the older person. Isolation increases the probability of abuse.
- Give contradictory versions of events concerning the elder adult.
- Be noncompliant with service providers in planning for the client's care.
- Be defensive when asked about the elder.

FACTORS LEADING TO ABUSE

History of Abuse

There is a relationship between the way the elderly person treated the caregiver and the way the caregiver treats the elderly person now.

- The mother maltreated the child, and the adult child may now abuse the mother.
- The wife who is the primary caregiver may maltreat the abusive spouse.

- The older person may physically abuse the caregiver, which is common among clients with Alzheimer's disease.

Changes in Living Situations

- The older person's growing frailty and dependence may cause him or her to move in with an adult child. This can cause hostility in the family created by the older person's presence.
- The elderly person may need to relocate because of physical limitations, creating a financial hardship on the adult child.

Stress of Caregiving

- The stress of being a caregiver is a significant risk factor in relation to abuse and neglect.
- Intense frustration and anger can lead to a range of abusive behaviors.
- Caregivers may be unaware of the demands of daily care for an older adult until the role begins. The greater the disability, the greater the risk for abuse.
- Most caregivers do not have the appropriate training. If not trained for dealing with difficult behaviors, caregivers can find themselves using physical force.
- The caregiver must learn how to balance the needs of the older person with his or her own needs to reduce feelings of hopelessness.
- The lack of available resources and assistance may increase the stress level of the caregiver.

Dependence

- The caregiver may be financially dependent on the older person and may become resentful.
- An impaired elder is dependent on the caregiver. The caregiver's loss of independence may lead to abusive behavior.

Emotional and Psychological Problems of the Caregiver

- The caregiver may have a preexisting mental illness.
- Abusers are more likely to use drugs or alcohol. This can lead to a greater chance of alcohol or drug abuse in an attempt to manage the stress.
- The caregiver may have low self-esteem because of being financially dependent on the older person.
- The caregiver may use violence to solve problems because of limited coping skills.

Lack of Respect for the Elderly

- Our society tends to celebrate the young and disregard older adults.
- Some cultures do not respect the wisdom of the elderly.

Religious or Cultural Beliefs

- Mistreatment of family members, especially women, is common in some cultures. Those who participate in these behaviors do not consider them abuse.
- In some cultures, women's basic rights are not honored, and older women in these cultures may not realize they are being abused. They probably could not go outside the family for help and may not be aware that help is available.

REPORTING ELDER ABUSE

- Each state designates who is mandated to report incidents of elder abuse. Adult Protective Services is the principal public agency responsible for both investigating reported cases of elder abuse and providing victims and their families with treatment and protective services.
- Contact your local Adult Protective Services for individual state information.
- Elder abuse can be a sensitive topic because of the rights of older Americans. This means that an elderly person:
  - may live in a self-destructive manner, as long as no crimes are committed and no one is harmed.
  - has the right to make decisions until he or she delegates responsibility to someone else or the court grants this responsibility to someone else.
  - has the right to confidentiality; personal information, including suspected abuse, may not be shared without consent.

(Insert your agency's policy regarding reporting abuse here.)

PREVENTING ELDER ABUSE

No one, at any age, should be subjected to violent, abusive, humiliating, or neglectful behavior. Because most abuse occurs in the home, it is important to educate the public about the special needs of the elderly and the risk factors for abuse.

Reasons Elder Abuse Is Not Reported

- What happens at home is "private."
- Outsiders may fail to intervene because "it is a family problem," "it is none of my business," or "it is just a misunderstanding."
- Older adults may be too ashamed and embarrassed to reveal abuse.
- The victims do not want others to know that such events occur in their families.

Educating People About Elder Abuse

People need to understand the:

- Signs of abuse.
- Causes of abuse.
- Stress of being a caregiver.

Respite Care

- Respite care is having someone else take care of the elderly person temporarily, which gives the caregiver a break from caring for the family member. The break can alleviate stress, which is a major risk factor for abuse.
- Respite can range from a few hours (the caregiver can go to the movies or have a date with spouse or children) to a few weeks (the caregiver can take a family vacation or a business trip).
- Caregivers of complete-care clients, such as those with Alzheimer's disease or other forms of dementia and the severely disabled, should use respite care as often as possible.

Assistive Programs and Support Services

Home Care Services

- Assist with activities of daily living.
- Perform nursing assessment.

Adult Day Care Programs

- Care for the elder during the day.
- Provide social outlets and respite for the caregiver.

Support Groups

- Help the caregiver by giving him or her a place to discuss problems.
- Provide a social forum for caregivers, in which families in similar circumstances can band together to share solutions and provide informal respite for each other.

Counseling

- Provides treatment to help cope with personal and family problems.
- Helps caregivers to find ways to solve problems and cope with stress.

Placement

- Includes long-term care facilities or adult foster-care programs, which may be the best option for the aging client.
- Helps to relieve stress, which may lead to abuse.

Instructor's version with answers for Handout 3-2

REAL-LIFE SCENARIO

A 68-year-old woman, who was wheelchair-bound from multiple sclerosis, asked her son and his family to move in with her to help with the household bills and to assist her. Within months, the son moved her to the small upstairs bedroom. This meant that she was totally dependent on her son for everything. As time went on, the family assisted less. If it were not for the HCA, the client would not get bathed or fed. The son and his family did not provide meals, medications, or any assistance with activities of daily living. The only time the family would see her is when they wanted her to sign her social security check. The client would call the home care agency daily because that was the only outside contact she had.

On many visits, the social worker, nurse, and HCA would discuss more accommodating living arrangements. The client stated that she was going to stay in her house and that it was not as bad as it seemed. There was nothing the health care team could do but to provide her with support and information.

Question 1. What types of elder abuse are described?

Answer: This scenario describes financial and emotional abuse and neglect.

Question 2. What can be done to educate the public about elder abuse?

Answer: The public should be educated about the signs of abuse, indicators of abuse, factors leading to abuse, and the stress of being a caregiver.

Question 3. Does the state have the right to remove the client from the home if she does not want to leave?

Answer: The elderly have the right to determine their affairs to the full extent of their ability as long as they are deemed competent. No one can force a competent adult to change the way she lives even if it threatens her health or safety. The client could not be legally moved because she was competent and chose to stay in the home.

GROUP ACTIVITY

1. Ask the audience to describe examples of elder abuse.
2. Have volunteers act out a skit involving elder abuse.
3. List ways to control anger and frustration to avoid abuse.
4. Discuss examples of spouse abuse.
   - The partner may embarrass the person in front of others.
   - The partner may belittle the person's accomplishments.
   - The partner may be contradicting to confuse the person.
   - The partner may isolate the person from loved ones.
   - The partner may make the person believe that he is not smart so that he does not make any decisions.
   - The partner may make the person perform acts that are demeaning.
   - The partner may prevent the person from leaving the house.
   - The partner may get angry if the person visits friends and family or talks to the opposite sex.
   - The partner may control all of the finances.
   - The partner may make the person believe one cannot exist without the other.
   - The partner may make the person feel that there is no way out.
   - The partner may treat the person roughly by grabbing, slapping, kicking, pinching, pushing, or shoving.
   - The partner may threaten the person verbally or with a weapon.
   - The partner may get angry without any cause.
   - The partner may physically force or intimidate the person to do something.
5. Discuss examples of the victim's reaction to abuse.
   - The victim may want to help the partner change the abusive behavior.
   - The victim may spend time trying to find ways not to make the partner angry.
   - The victim may do what the partner wants rather than what he or she wants, out of fear.
   - The victim may stay with the partner only because of fear.

 RESOURCES

Administration on Aging
http://www.aoa.dhhs.gov

The National Center on Elder Abuse
http://www.elderabusecenter.org

National Child Abuse Hotline
1-800-4-A-CHILD (800-422-4453)
TDD: 1-800-2-A-CHILD

The National Clearinghouse on Child Abuse and Neglect
http://www.calib.com/nccanch/statutes.htm

The National Council on Child Abuse and Family Violence
http://www.nccafv.org

National Domestic Violence Hotline
800-799-SAFE (7233), or 800-787-3224 (TDD)
24 hours a day

Nationwide Eldercare Locator toll-free number
1-800-677-1116

U.S. Department of Health and Human Services
http://www.acf.dhhs.gov/

U.S. Department of Justice, Office of Justice Programs Web site
http://www.ojp.usdoj.gov/vawo/welcome.htm

REFERENCES

Administration on Aging. (1998, September). *National elder abuse incidence study.* Retrieved December 19, 2000, from http://www.aoa.gov/abuse/reprot/Fdesign.htm.

The Administration for Children and Families. (1997). *Child maltreatment 1997: Reports from the states to the National Child Abuse and Neglect Data System.* Retrieved December 2, 2000, from http://www.acf.dhhs.gov/programs/cb.

Allan, M. (1998). Elder abuse: A challenge for home care nurses. *Home Healthcare Nurse, 16*(2), 103–110.

Cyphers, G. C. (1999). Out of the shadows: Elder abuse and neglect. *Policy & Practice of Public Human Services, 57*(3), 25–30. Retrieved December 5, 2000, from http://proquest.umi.com/pqdweb.

Decalmer, P., & Glendenning, F. (Eds.). (1997). *The mistreatment of elderly people.* London: Sage.

Gaudin, J. M., Jr. (1993, April). *Child neglect: A guide for intervention.* For U.S. Department of Health and Human Services, Administration for Children and Families, Administration on Children, Youth and Families. National Center on Child Abuse and Neglect. Washington, DC: Westover Consultants.

Korfmacher, J. (1998). *Emotional neglect: Being hurt by what is not there.* Chicago: National Committee to Prevent Child Abuse.

Prevent Child Abuse America. *Ten ways to help prevent child abuse.* Retrieved December 12, 2000, from http://www.preventchildabuse.org.

Prevent Child Abuse America. *Twelve alternatives to lashing out at your child.* Retrieved December 12, 2000, from http://www.preventchildabuse.org.

State Statutes Project. (2000, May). *Definitions of child abuse and neglect.* Retrieved December 12, 2000, from http://www.calib.com/nccanch/statutes.htm.

State Statutes Project. (2000, May). *Mandatory reporters of child abuse and neglect.* Retrieved December 12, 2000, from http://www.calib.com/nccanch/statutes.htm.

Tatara, T., & Kuzmeskus, L. M. (1997, November). *Elder abuse information series.* Retrieved December 19, 2000, from http://www.elderabusecenter.org.

U.S. Department of Health and Human Services, Administration on Children, Youth and Families. (2001). *Child maltreatment 1999.* Washington, DC: U.S. Government Printing Office.

Wieland, D. (2000). Abuse of older persons: An overview. *Holistic Nursing Practice, 14*(4), 40–50. Retrieved December 5, 2000, from http://proquest.umi.com/pqdweb.

Name _____ Date _____
Program/Course _____ Instructor's Name _____

ABUSE
Pre/Post Test

1. According to CAPTA, child abuse is defined as:
   a. failure to act on the part of the caretaker resulting in death, serious physical or emotional harm, or sexual exploitation.
   b. the victim must be less than 18 years old.
   c. an act or failure to act that causes imminent risk of serious harm.
   d. all of the above.

2. Signs of physical abuse include:
   a. bruises in various stages of healing.
   b. malnourishment.
   c. inappropriate clothing.
   d. missed doctor's appointments.

3. Which of the following is an example of financial abuse?
   a. inability to manage personal finances
   b. deceiving an older person into signing documents
   c. failing to pay bills
   d. all of the above

4. Define self-neglect.
   a. any refusal or failure of a caregiver to provide basic needs to an older person
   b. any refusal or failure of a caregiver to provide basic needs to an older person, excluding those who are mentally competent
   c. any behavior that threatens an older person's health or safety because of his or her own limitations
   d. any behavior that threatens an older person's health or safety because of his or her own limitations, excluding clients who are mentally competent

5. Intimidation is a form of domestic violence. Which of the following is an example of intimidation?
   a. repeatedly insulting the partner
   b. using physical harm as a method of control
   c. using looks, actions, or gestures to control the partner's behavior
   d. controlling all finances and preventing the partner from getting a job

Handout **3-1**

Name _____ Date _____

Program/Course _____ Instructor's Name _____

REAL-LIFE SCENARIO

A 68-year-old woman, who was wheelchair-bound from multiple sclerosis, asked her son and his family to move in with her to help with the household bills and to assist her. Within months, the son moved her to the small upstairs bedroom. This meant that she was totally dependent on her son for everything. As time went on, the family assisted less. If it were not for the HCA, the client would not get bathed or fed. The son and his family did not provide meals, medications, or any assistance with activities of daily living. The only time the family would see her is when they wanted her to sign her social security check. The client would call the home-care agency daily because that was the only outside contact she had.

On many visits, the social worker, nurse, and HCA would discuss more accommodating living arrangements. The client stated that she was going to stay in her house and that it was not as bad as it seemed. There was nothing the health care team could do but to provide her with support and information.

Question 1. What types of elder abuse are described?

Question 2. What can be done to educate the public about elder abuse?

Question 3. Does the state have the right to remove the client from the home if she does not want to leave?

Handout **3-2**

ABUSE

Signs of physical abuse

- **Trauma markings on back or abdomen**
- **Bruises in various stages of healing**
- **Burns**
- **Fractures and head injuries in young children**
- **Human bites**

Signs of emotional abuse

- Extreme behaviors/low self-esteem
- Overly friendly to strangers
- Delays in physical/emotional development
- Difficulty with close relationships
- Problems in school

Signs of sexual abuse

- **Changes in behavior/very secretive**
- **Pain when walking/sitting**
- **Poor appearance**
- **Inappropriate sexual behavior**
- **Frightened by physical contact**
- **Pregnancy or STD at a young age**

Signs of neglect

- Generally poor hygiene
- Problems in school
- Behavioral concerns
- Problems with relationships
- Alcohol or drug use

Tips to control anger and frustration

- Use relaxation techniques.
- Take a "time-out."
- Find a respite.
- Call 1-800-CHILDREN.

Types of domestic violence

- **Physical abuse**
- **Sexual abuse**
- **Psychological abuse**
  - **Verbal abuse**
  - **Intimidation/isolation**

Categories of elder abuse

- **Domestic elder abuse**
- **Institutional elder abuse**
- **Self-neglect or self-abuse**

Signs of physical abuse of the elderly

- Poor general physical appearance
- Changes in behavior
- Untreated injuries
- Injuries in various stages of healing
- Signs of being restrained

Signs of emotional abuse of the elderly

- Emotionally upset or agitated
- Withdrawn/noncommunicative/nonresponsive
- Difficulty sleeping
- Unusual behavior
- Symptoms improve when not in the care of abuser

Signs of sexual abuse of the elderly

- Injuries around the breasts or genital area
- STDs without explanation
- Vaginal or anal bleeding
- Torn garments
- Pain when walking or sitting

Signs of financial abuse of the elderly

- **Unauthorized changes in assets/will**
- **Misuse of power of attorney**
- **Valuables disappearing**
- **Uninvolved relatives claiming rights**

Neglect of the elderly

- Caregiver neglect
- Self-neglect
- Abandonment

LICENSE AGREEMENT FOR THOMSON DELMAR LEARNING

Set Up Instructions:
1. Insert disc into CD-ROM player. The program should start up automatically. If it does not, go to step 2.
2. From My Computer, double click the icon for the CD drive.
3. Double click the *start.exe* file to start the program.

System Requirements:
- Operating system: Microsoft® Windows™ 98, Me, NT 4.0, 2000, XP, or newer
- Processor: Pentium (120 MHz) processor or faster
- Memory: 24 MB
- Hard disk space: 16 MB
- Monitor: VGA-compatible color
- CD-ROM drive: 4x

Microsoft® is a registered trademark and Windows® and Windows NT® are trademarks of Microsoft Corporation.

End User License Agreement

IMPORTANT! READ CAREFULLY: This End User License Agreement ("Agreement") sets forth the conditions by which Thomson Delmar Learning, a division of Thomson Learning Inc. ("Thomson") will make electronic access to the Thomson Delmar Learning-owned licensed content and associated media, software, documentation, printed materials, and electronic documentation contained in this package and/or made available to you via this product (the "Licensed Content"), available to you (the "End User"). BY CLICKING THE "I ACCEPT" BUTTON AND/OR OPENING THIS PACKAGE, YOU ACKNOWLEDGE THAT YOU HAVE READ ALL OF THE TERMS AND CONDITIONS, AND THAT YOU AGREE TO BE BOUND BY ITS TERMS, CONDITIONS, AND ALL APPLICABLE LAWS AND REGULATIONS GOVERNING THE USE OF THE LICENSED CONTENT.

1.0 SCOPE OF LICENSE

1.1 <u>Licensed Content.</u> The Licensed Content may contain portions of modifiable content ("Modifiable Content") and content which may not be modified or otherwise altered by the End User ("Non-Modifiable Content"). For purposes of this Agreement, Modifiable Content and Non-Modifiable Content may be collectively referred to herein as the "Licensed Content." All Licensed Content shall be considered Non-Modifiable Content, unless such Licensed Content is presented to the End User in a modifiable format and it is clearly indicated that modification of the Licensed Content is permitted.

1.2 Subject to the End User's compliance with the terms and conditions of this Agreement, Thomson Delmar Learning hereby grants the End User, a nontransferable, nonexclusive, limited right to access and view a single copy of the Licensed Content on a single personal computer system for noncommercial, internal, personal use only. The End User shall not (i) reproduce, copy, modify (except in the case of Modifiable Content), distribute, display, transfer, sublicense, prepare derivative work(s) based on, sell, exchange, barter or transfer, rent, lease, loan, resell, or in any other manner exploit the Licensed Content; (ii) remove, obscure, or alter any notice of Thomson Delmar Learning's intellectual property rights present on or in the Licensed Content, including, but not limited to, copyright, trademark, and/or patent notices; or (iii) disassemble, decompile, translate, reverse engineer, or otherwise reduce the Licensed Content.

2.0 TERMINATION

2.1 Thomson Delmar Learning may at any time (without prejudice to its other rights or remedies) immediately terminate this Agreement and/or suspend access to some or all of the Licensed Content, in the event that the End User does not comply with any of the terms and conditions of this Agreement. In the event of such termination by Thomson Delmar Learning, the End User shall immediately return any and all copies of the Licensed Content to Thomson Delmar Learning.

3.0 PROPRIETARY RIGHTS

3.1 The End User acknowledges that Thomson Delmar Learning owns all rights, title and interest, including, but not limited to all copyright rights therein, in and to the Licensed Content, and that the End User shall not take any action inconsistent with such ownership. The Licensed Content is protected by U.S., Canadian and other applicable copyright laws and by international treaties, including the Berne Convention and the Universal Copyright Convention. Nothing contained in this Agreement shall be construed as granting the End User any ownership rights in or to the Licensed Content.

3.2 Thomson Delmar Learning reserves the right at any time to withdraw from the Licensed Content any item or part of an item for which it no longer retains the right to publish, or which it has reasonable grounds to believe infringes copyright or is defamatory, unlawful, or otherwise objectionable.

4.0 PROTECTION AND SECURITY

4.1 The End User shall use its best efforts and take all reasonable steps to safeguard its copy of the Licensed Content to ensure that no unauthorized reproduction, publication, disclosure, modification, or distribution of the Licensed Content, in whole or in part, is made. To the extent that the End User becomes aware of any such unauthorized use of the Licensed Content, the End User shall immediately notify Thomson Delmar Learning. Notification of such violations may be made by sending an e-mail to delmarhelp@thomson.com.

5.0 MISUSE OF THE LICENSED PRODUCT

5.1 In the event that the End User uses the Licensed Content in violation of this Agreement, Thomson Delmar Learning shall have the option of electing liquidated damages, which shall include all profits generated by the End User's use of the Licensed Content plus interest computed at the maximum rate permitted by law and all legal fees and other expenses incurred by Thomson Delmar Learning in enforcing its rights, plus penalties.

6.0 FEDERAL GOVERNMENT CLIENTS

6.1 Except as expressly authorized by Thomson Delmar Learning, Federal Government clients obtain only the rights specified in this Agreement and no other rights. The Government acknowledges that (i) all software and related documentation incorporated in the Licensed Content is existing commercial computer software within the meaning of FAR 27.405(b)(2); and (2) all other data delivered in whatever form, is limited rights data within the meaning of FAR 27.401. The restrictions in this section are acceptable as consistent with the Government's need for software and other data under this Agreement.

7.0 DISCLAIMER OF WARRANTIES AND LIABILITIES

7.1 Although Thomson Delmar Learning believes the Licensed Content to be reliable, Thomson Delmar Learning does not guarantee or warrant (i) any information or materials contained in or produced by the Licensed Content, (ii) the accuracy, completeness or reliability of the Licensed Content, or (iii) that the Licensed Content is free from errors or other material defects. THE LICENSED PRODUCT IS PROVIDED "AS IS," WITHOUT ANY WARRANTY OF ANY KIND AND THOMSON DELMAR LEARNING DISCLAIMS ANY AND ALL WARRANTIES, EXPRESSED OR IMPLIED, INCLUDING, WITHOUT LIMITATION, WARRANTIES OF MERCHANTABILITY OR FITNESS OR A PARTICULAR PURPOSE. IN NO EVENT SHALL THOMSON DELMAR LEARNING BE LIABLE FOR: INDIRECT, SPECIAL, PUNITIVE OR CONSEQUENTIAL DAMAGES INCLUDING FOR LOST PROFITS, LOST DATA, OR OTHERWISE. IN NO EVENT SHALL THOMSON DELMAR LEARNING'S AGGREGATE LIABILITY HEREUNDER, WHETHER ARISING IN CONTRACT, TORT, STRICT LIABILITY OR OTHERWISE, EXCEED THE AMOUNT OF FEES PAID BY THE END USER HEREUNDER FOR THE LICENSE OF THE LICENSED CONTENT.

8.0 GENERAL

8.1 <u>Entire Agreement.</u> This Agreement shall constitute the entire Agreement between the Parties and supercedes all prior Agreements and understandings oral or written relating to the subject matter hereof.

8.2 <u>Enhancements/Modifications of Licensed Content.</u> From time to time, and in Thomson Delmar Learning's sole discretion, Thomson Delmar Learning may advise the End User of updates, upgrades, enhancements and/or improvements to the Licensed Content, and may permit the End User to access and use, subject to the terms and conditions of this Agreement, such modifications, upon payment of prices as may be established by Thomson Delmar Learning.

8.3 <u>No Export.</u> The End User shall use the Licensed Content solely in the United States and shall not transfer or export, directly or indirectly, the Licensed Content outside the United States.

8.4 <u>Severability.</u> If any provision of this Agreement is invalid, illegal, or unenforceable under any applicable statute or rule of law, the provision shall be deemed omitted to the extent that it is invalid, illegal, or unenforceable. In such a case, the remainder of the Agreement shall be construed in a manner as to give greatest effect to the original intention of the parties hereto.

8.5 <u>Waiver.</u> The waiver of any right or failure of either party to exercise in any respect any right provided in this Agreement in any instance shall not be deemed to be a waiver of such right in the future or a waiver of any other right under this Agreement.

8.6 <u>Choice of Law/Venue.</u> This Agreement shall be interpreted, construed, and governed by and in accordance with the laws of the State of New York, applicable to contracts executed and to be wholly preformed therein, without regard to its principles governing conflicts of law. Each party agrees that any proceeding arising out of or relating to this Agreement or the breach or threatened breach of this Agreement may be commenced and prosecuted in a court in the State and County of New York. Each party consents and submits to the nonexclusive personal jurisdiction of any court in the State and County of New York in respect of any such proceeding.

8.7 <u>Acknowledgment.</u> By opening this package and/or by accessing the Licensed Content on this Web site, THE END USER ACKNOWLEDGES THAT IT HAS READ THIS AGREEMENT, UNDERSTANDS IT, AND AGREES TO BE BOUND BY ITS TERMS AND CONDITIONS. IF YOU DO NOT ACCEPT THESE TERMS AND CONDITIONS, YOU MUST NOT ACCESS THE LICENSED CONTENT AND RETURN THE LICENSED PRODUCT TO DELMAR LEARNING (WITHIN 30 CALENDAR DAYS OF THE END USER'S PURCHASE) WITH PROOF OF PAYMENT ACCEPTABLE TO THOMSON DELMAR LEARNING, FOR A CREDIT OR A REFUND. Should the End User have any questions/comments regarding this Agreement, please contact Thomson Delmar Learning at delmarhelp@thomson.com.